integrative medicine for
BINGE EATING

A comprehensive guide to the New Hope Model for the elimination of binge eating and food cravings

James Greenblatt, MD
and Virginia Ross-Taylor, PhD

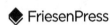 FriesenPress

Suite 300 - 990 Fort St
Victoria, BC, V8V 3K2
Canada

www.friesenpress.com

Copyright © 2019 by James Greenblatt
First Edition — 2019

All rights reserved.

No part of this publication may be reproduced in any form, or by any means, electronic or mechanical, including photocopying, recording, or any information browsing, storage, or retrieval system, without permission in writing from FriesenPress.

ISBN
978-1-5255-4192-6 (Hardcover)
978-1-5255-4193-3 (Paperback)
978-1-5255-4194-0 (eBook)

1. SELF-HELP, EATING DISORDERS & BODY IMAGE

Distributed to the trade by The Ingram Book Company

TABLE OF CONTENTS

Foreword by Stuart L. Koman, PhD ... v
Foreword Ralph Carson, LD, RD, PhD ... ix
Introduction: Getting Off the Roller Coaster ... xiii

Part I. The Roller-Coaster Ride of Binge Eating and Food Addiction ... **1**
1 The New Hope: Restoring Control ... 3
2 Addicted to Food: My Dopamine Made Me Do It ... 17
3 The Appetite Gone Wild: Many Forms of Disordered Eating ... 27
4 You Are Extraordinary: The Genetics of Appetite and Weight Control ... 35
5 Comprehensive Evaluations for Appetite Control ... 47
6 Food Addiction: The Science of Sugar ... 57
7 Food Addiction: The Chemistry of Dairy and Wheat ... 69

Part II. Personalized Nutritional Supplements for Binge Eating and Food Addiction ... **79**
8 Laboratory Evaluations for Individualized Nutritional Support ... 81
9 Controlling Appetite with Amino Acid Supplements ... 103
10 Controlling Appetite with Vitamin and Mineral Supplements ... 127

Part III. Medications for Binge Eating and Food Addiction ... **149**
11 Controlling Appetite with Medications ... 151

Part IV. Lifestyle Changes for Binge Eating and Food Addiction   **171**

12 What Not to Eat: High Fructose Corn Syrup
   & Artificial Sweeteners   173
13 What Not to Eat: Monosodium Glutamate   183
14 Controlling Appetite with an UN-Diet   193
15 Rediscovering Hope through Therapy   203
16 Mastering the Balance of Movement and Sleep   217

Part V. Your New Hope   **229**
17 Survival of the Fattest   231

About the Authors   **237**

References   **239**

FOREWORD

By Stuart L. Koman, PhD

America is obsessed with food and weight; the rest of the world is following close behind. We are inundated daily with news and information from TV, magazines, electronic media and mostly each other about what we're eating, what celebrity is "rocking" the bikini in Maui, how to exercise and what foods contain what nutrients and antioxidants to save us from Alzheimer's or diabetes. For many people, the ideal and quest for thinness and body perfection trump any other personal goal or life direction. And all of this happens against a backdrop of out-of-control eating that has seen more individuals slip into the categories of overweight, obese and even "super" obese than at any other time in the known history of the world. If you're a person who does not fall into one of these three camps, you are now officially part of the minority.

What is happening here? While much has been written describing the state of affairs, we have no answers, certainly, at the societal level as to what is fueling this situation. Various physical and behavioral scientists and theorists have blamed everything from the emergence of processed foods and food additives to wheat and dairy products to a conspiracy of the entertainment and fashion industries to explain these phenomena. I think it is not being overly dramatic to say that the very well-being of the human race is now dependent on reversing this trend, but I see no emerging clarity in the near term and very little collaboration across disciplinary lines in the scientific community to figure it out. We would do well to emulate the genetic researchers, biochemists and doctors who after many years of working in isolation to find the cure for cancer began working as teams. The last fifteen years has witnessed an explosion of effective treatments for many types of cancers.

These issues reach crisis proportion for those of us in the medical and behavioral health field when we are confronted with real live people, our patients, who are suffering and beseeching us to provide a rational road to recovery or at least a modicum of hope for the future. Too often, the approach suggested depends entirely upon what door you enter: if you consult a surgeon, you'll likely get surgery; a psychiatrist, you'll likely get medication; a nutritionist, you'll likely get a meal plan; a psychologist, you'll likely get therapy. There is nothing inherently wrong with any of these approaches. They all can and have been helpful for many people. But none of them are helpful for everyone and many of them seem to work best in combination with one or more of the others. But how is the average person to know how to figure out what he or she individually needs to do?

Returning to the example of cancer treatment, great progress has been made by learning how to target specific types of the disease. Whereas 50 years ago, there was just the "Big C", now we have research, clinical trials and specialty clinics for dozens of expressions of the disease. Melanoma is treated differently than lymphoma or leukemia. We do not yet have near the level of expertise or research that allows us to make the same claim about eating disorders, but 30 years of clinical experience with eating and other mental diseases tells me that there are many routes to similar configurations of symptoms that we classify into diagnostic groups known as anorexia, bulimia, binge eating and obesity. In this case, diagnosis does little to determine a successful course of treatment and may actually hinder its development if the practitioner rigidly ascribes to a particular approach that is more dependent on his or her training and less dependent on the unique aspects of the patient sitting in front of him or her.

This book makes an immediate contribution to the field in two related ways. The first advancement is in the recognition of each individual's unique biology as the primary determinant of the treatment approach.

A careful laboratory assessment at the beginning of treatment is critical in beginning the process that leads to a targeted treatment plan. To this excellent start, I would add a similar assessment of each individual's unique psychology because no treatment will work without the patient's buy in and follow through; motivation and treatment compliance are critical factors in determining how to proceed clinically.

The integrative approach presented here is the big step forward and, hopefully, a beginning to the end of the craziness that has ruled the field for too long. While this is by no means a treatment cookbook with tried and true recipes (food analogies are hard to get way from in this culture) for weight loss, it will serve well as an effective organizer and source of information for individuals who are trying to get a grip and find a starting point for addressing their uncomfortable relationship with food.

It is critical, as Dr. Greenblatt points out, to truly assess and understand the drivers of disordered eating: individual vulnerability to specific foods, undiagnosed psychiatric conditions and major disruption of the brain reward mechanism are all possible culprits that can easily hijack a person's psychology, sense of self and ultimately his or her prospects for a full and meaningful life.

Stuart L. Koman, PhD
Founder and Chief Executive of Walden Behavioral Care

FOREWORD

By Ralph Carson, LD, RD, PhD

There is a fundamental fallacy that weight loss diets have the miraculous ability to transform any individual to the promised land of a yet-to-be determined "ideal weight." Historically, since 1856 beginning with the Banting Diet, diets have failed repeatedly as evidenced by the paucity of those who are capable of reaching that nebulous magic number on the scale and maintaining it long term. The outcome should not be surprising in that there are thousands of diets composed of actually the same three macronutrients: carbohydrates, fats and protein.

So if diets did not work 40 years ago, there is no reason we should assume they will work in today's world of an overabundance of highly palatable foods and inactive lifestyles. It is equally ludicrous to surmise that exercising alone would contribute significantly to fat reduction. Research supports the mathematics of caloric expenditure, which calculates exercise as an inefficient modality to reduce one's size. Yes, there are individuals, call them "outliers" if you will, who can weather the pseudo-starvation and draconian exercise necessary to achieve a desirable size and weight. This number is discouragingly low and has remained such over decades of dieting and exercise attempts. And what is even more disheartening is that even upon achieving newfound thinness, the achievement does not guarantee happiness.

James Greenblatt, MD

It is a breath of fresh air that a highly respected veteran in the field of eating disorders, Dr. James Greenblatt, is addressing this chronic and complex condition of size with a contemporary scheme and scientific insight. This book, *Integrative Medicine for Binge Eating*, recognizes that we should honor human diversity and realize that every person is unique. As such, there is a demand for a personalized plan that assesses hormonal, genetic, spiritual, nutritional, behavioral and neurological differences to combat the plethora of challenges involved in recovery. The American population is inundated with information regarding what they should do nutritionally and physically, but that has not stopped the ever-increasing rise in health concerns associated with adiposity and the pathological dieting that breeds eating disorders.

Regulating appetite is a major theme in the battle to control what goes into our bodies. It is not a simple matter of homeostatic control often referred to as "eat when you are hungry and stop when you are full." We all have become over-stimulated by a commercial environment of highly processed foods designed to trick us into eating beyond the point of fullness. The hedonics (smell, taste, mouth feel and appearance of food) are now the driving force behind what determines if one is satisfied and consequently brings a meal to an end. With a motivational brain circuit that is programmed to seek pleasure, it is reasonable to make comparisons as to how highly palatable foods share similar pathways with addictive drugs. Repeated use and overconsumption can alter brain chemistry and wiring so that it creates a state of unmanageable urges. Even in spite of negative consequences, these powerful cravings are impossible to resist regardless of how much willpower one intrinsically possesses.

Layered onto the strong command of the pleasure center dictating what we should eat, there lies an urgency and persistent need to quiet our emotions. It has long been known in animals and recently shown in human studies that carbohydrates act on serotonin to calm or numb our various depressed mood states. In an alternative neurological pathway, fatty acids can quiet the anxiety center or amygdala. Yet the stress of dieting, pain of exercise and frustration of poor outcomes—along with the shame of repeated failure—only adds fuel to the emotional roller coaster. Left unchecked, success is transient because the underlying triggers continue to kindle in the deep confines of the midbrain or limbic system.

The intrusive thoughts we possess soon become desires and proceed to urges and ultimately cravings. Eventually we can become obsessed, so these cravings become unmanageable and the behavior turns into a compulsion. To combat this conflict within the mind calls for a knowledgeable and skilled therapeutic team experienced in psychotherapy, mindfulness and medications. The medications can make our thought processes more flexible and capable of changing. Certain pharmaceuticals act as a catalyst to speed up the transition and allow for self-control to take over. Medications can also ease the journey through the uncomfortable symptoms and make permanent recovery more likely to occur. Psychotherapy will stimulate new brain cell growth and rewire circuits as we challenge dysfunctional behaviors and substitute them with more constructive behaviors. Through habit change we will learn to incorporate the parts of our brain that serve as the wise advocate. And mindfulness practices will allow us to change the way we think by being in the present and non-judgmental as we sit with those intrusive thoughts. Through this technique that requires practice and regularity, we will move through the problem instead of allowing it to persist and control our lives.

In treating the problem at hand, the wise advice proposed by this book lies in reestablishing balance. This approach is multifaceted and respects each individual's differences and previous experiences. Co-occurring conditions (attention-deficit hyperactivity disorder, obsessive-compulsive disorder, post-traumatic stress disorder, anxiety disorder, depression, eating disorders, etc.) must be identified and treated appropriately. To disregard these entities will provide only a partial fix that could reignite or exacerbate a recurrence of the problem in the future. Highly trained therapists are needed to identify these conditions and work out a treatment plan that coincides with the goals set forth for recovery.

Fundamentally, the brains of those being treated have been depleted. This demands not only replenishing brain stores, but also preventing further deterioration. Elements for regeneration of neurons and rewiring of circuits include quality nutrients and often evidenced-based use of supplements. At the same time, the individual may need to omit the destructive intake of items that in specific instances could cause further harm and deterioration (gluten, casein, monosodium glutamate, artificial sweeteners, high fructose corn syrup). This healing process is orchestrated by growth hormones that are provided during sleep. Quality sleep is necessary then to insure that healing and repair take place. To make all this happen efficiently and expediently requires the addition of growth factors or "miracle grow for the brain." It has been firmly established that the leading contributors to enhancing such chemicals as brain derived neurotrophic factor are exercise, meditation and cognitive behavioral therapy.

The dimension I appreciate most in this exposé on appetite control is the emphasis on the importance of engaging in proper assessments, labs and testing. It is critical to identify the underlying problems and to do so in a thorough, well-designed and complete fashion. The analyzing of nutritional, metabolic and biochemical needs should be assigned to a competent collection of trained healthcare professionals who are familiar with the individuality of the patient. The overall scheme falls under the heading of integrative medicine where traditional and complementary techniques are employed in tandem.

Recovery from any eating disorder ultimately lies with managing appetite, urges and fears. There has long been support for treatment plans that incorporate body, mind and spirit in order to access complete recovery. These chapters effectively educate one on the integrative approach to optimize brain health and provide the tools necessary to tailor it to each individual's needs. It is not a journey one should take on or assume he or she can accomplish on his or her own—one should seek the aid of an experienced professional and integrated team. With proper assessments and evaluation and a healthy dose of self-efficacy, recovery will become a reality and consequently one's life will flourish.

Ralph E. Carson, LD, RD, PhD
Senior Clinical and Research Advisor, Eating Recovery Centers
Author of *The Brain Fix: What's the Matter with Your Gray Matter*

INTRODUCTION: GETTING OFF THE ROLLER COASTER

It has been said that the world is divided into two kinds of people: those who live to eat and those who eat to live. That is, those who are passionate about food and those who like food but who eat primarily for the sustenance that allows them to live their lives.

The truth is, the world is much more complex than that. There is a third category: individuals for whom food is something other than enjoyment or sustenance; people for whom food is a cruel taskmaster that dominates their life day-to-day and often minute-to-minute. This scenario might sound familiar to you. Although you might feel completely isolated and alone, millions of people struggle with a similar unhealthy, unhappy, and unsatisfying relationship with food.

Like all unsuccessful relationships, your relationship with food is complex and complicated. It is not your "fault." Understanding exactly what has gone wrong in your relationship and, more importantly, understanding how to make it "right" again is what you will discover in this book.

Historically, our relationship with food has rested on the balance between our need to eat and the availability of food: the biological imperative to eat—hunger—and the physical ability to satisfy that imperative. The interplay between hunger and satisfaction is "appetite."

Appetite, at least in theory, is an internal guide that plots the path of when, what and how much we should eat. Like all our physiological systems, our appetite is best suited for the world in which our ancestors lived, a world of feast and famine. When food was scarce, our appetite was "on low", telling our bodies that little food was required. When food was plentiful, our appetites naturally amped up to allow us to take advantage of the relative bounty.

For many people living in this dawn of the twenty-first century, particularly those of us in first-world or westernized countries, food is always plentiful. There are no caloric "lean times." Our appetite, that trusty guide that served our ancestors so well in times past, is now out of sync with the reality of our modern lives. Rather than an aide in our survival, it has become a subversive enemy, undermining our good health and well-being.

It needn't be that way. Appetite is still one of the most important clues about what is happening in your body. It continues to perform the function that it always did—determining what you need to keep going and therefore when to start and stop eating.

That, ultimately, is what appetite does: it guides you by acting as the "stop" and "go" lights that regulate and temper your hunger. But stopping is not only a function of the lights but also of you in control of the car. The balance between appetite, hunger and eating depends a great deal on you.

Over the course of this book, you will learn to rebuild a good relationship with your appetite, getting to know your body's cues and signals, reset its chemistry and rediscover the most important element of any relationship—trust.

If the difference between "appetite" and "hunger" seems like splitting hairs to you right now, don't worry. In many ways, the two feel the same. They are the fraternal twins of diet, closely related, always intertwined, but still very distinct.

In fact, they are very different processes. Hunger is the need for food; appetite is the desire for food. Appetite exists so that you will find food attractive when it is available. That is, during those times of plenty, you will want to eat. Appetite is what causes you to salivate when you thumb through the pages of *Bon Appétit*. Appetite is what causes you to daydream about warm chocolate chip cookies, ice cream or shrimp scampi. It is desire and passion. It is a psychological, sensory process that triggers a physiological response.

Hunger, on the other hand, is a physical reaction that involves chemical changes in the body. It is an instinctive protective response that ensures the organism gets enough energy to fuel the body to function properly. The disconnect between hunger and appetite is the ticket onto the roller-coaster ride of disordered eating. This disconnect is repeated in slightly different configurations in millions of Americans. Although the individual journey differs for every person, many who struggle with disordered eating relate to the image of the roller coaster, and maybe you are one of them.

The roller-coaster ride of restricting, bingeing and chronic self-blame is never ending. There is the stretch of time when the car inches upward, when you feel a sense of progress. But then, without warning, you spiral downward in a great rush, having lost all sense of control. You crave, you eat, you binge. That momentary sense of calm and peace is once again overshadowed by shame and guilt.

While a roller-coaster ride may be a thrill to seek out at an amusement park, it is not a pleasant or useful way to live. No one chooses a pattern of disordered eating that damages health, self-esteem and personal relationships. So how do you get off the roller coaster? Based on more than thirty years of clinical experience, I have devised a program to help you get back on track. This program is an answer to binge eating disorder.

As obesity and the related health problems are now part of the national conversation, answers are now offered everywhere. Perhaps it is easier to talk first about proposed solutions that don't work. Adopting the latest new diet will not get you off the roller coaster. More than twenty-six million diet books are purchased in the U.S. in a given year. Inevitably, more will be rolled out the next year. This is because all the previously published diets ultimately fail to work on a lasting basis. People remain desperate for a solution to their struggles with food, and they still hold out hope that the next new diet book will offer the answer. But diets do not work over time. Countless studies show that while many individuals can successfully lose pounds on diets, the pounds return once there is an inevitable lapse. You cannot be vigilant about every morsel you take at every meal for the rest of your life. Even during the weeks of relative success, life becomes a tortured regimen. According to psychologists, even when people successfully follow a diet, they experience cravings for food at a much higher rate than non-dieters. And the constant calculation required to determine calorie counts and portion sizes takes away energy and concentration from enjoying both food and life itself.

If diets and diet books do not help, the medical culture has not helped either. "Just do it," counsels many a healthcare provider, echoing the words of the Nike commercial. Unfortunately, this well-intentioned advice will likely make you feel worse, not only about your weight but also about your lack of willpower.

In August 2013, Iris Higgins, a former weight loss consultant, wrote a courageous open apology to all her former clients for years of advice that she now believes was wrong. In her letter she apologized for putting clients on restricted calorie diets, for ignoring the need to check thyroid levels and for gluten sensitivity, for failing to recognize that weight loss plans do not solve the problem of a woman who hates her body for the fat that does not exist. Ms. Higgins and the weight loss company she worked for were not alone in selling out clients, she says now. "It was the doctors and registered dieticians on the medical advisory board. It was the media and magazines confirming what I was telling my patients." She now expresses heartfelt regret: "I helped you lose weight and then gain it back, so that you thought we were the solution and you were the failure. You became a repeat client and we kept you in the game."

As Iris Higgins and many in the medical profession now see, the way to get off the roller coaster of disordered eating is not through strict adherence to the latest weight loss program. The reason? Disordered eating is caused by *biology*, not by a deficit in will or character. Disordered eating is often caused by addiction to food. Eating foods high in sugar wreaks havoc with the body's natural systems of craving and reward, skewing the functioning of neurotransmitters, the chemical messengers in the brain. The food acts upon the part of the brain that makes you feel good, the center of pleasure and reward. Over time, and with the right biochemical vulnerability, the brain adapts to and compensates for the artificial revving up. Reacting to the sugar assault, it works overtime to restore equilibrium by decreasing the release of dopamine – a neurotransmitter heavily involved in reward-motivated behavior - leaving pleasure and reward circuits depleted. Without dopamine, the brain depends increasingly on an artificial stimulus to feel normal.

For many of you struggling with disordered eating, the dopamine cycle goes haywire in the same way it responds to alcohol in alcoholics. Both alcohol and food cues stimulate the reward circuitry in the brain. On a brain scan, the brain lights up in response to a food cue in the same way it lights up in response to the cue of alcohol. The part that lights up is the amygdala, a primitive region of the brain connected to pleasure that exerts its influence outside our conscious control. Because it is a deep, unconscious process, it is beyond the control of willpower.

This link between what we know about addiction and disordered eating has powerful implications. First, researchers have long been aware that addiction to alcohol is based on biochemical processes; it is a disease and not a moral failing. Similarly, disordered eating is not your fault! Secondly, there is a body of scientific literature about the biology of addiction that offers insight to those who wish to understand the mechanisms involved in addiction to food. From the rat studies alone, the evidence is convincing: a rat hooked on sugar will continue to push the food release lever in its cage even after its body swells to twice its normal size.

In this book, I have attempted to integrate insights from different fields of medicine and psychiatry as they relate to disordered eating. After more than 30 years in practice, I am convinced of the direct influences of what we eat and how we digest food on our behaviors and our feelings. This book explores the complex landscape of disordered eating and the tools now available to treat and to prevent it.

To be sure, our environment challenges those who want to get off the roller coaster. Television abounds with advertisements encouraging us to reward ourselves with sugary treats. Fast-food restaurants lure us with billboards featuring juicy cheeseburgers and milkshakes, and supermarket shelves offer attractively packaged processed foods. We have only to remember the tobacco industry's long campaign to keep us in the dark about the addictive potential of tobacco to recognize that the food industry will also fight hard with ever more attractive marketing strategies. Not only is access to food everywhere, we are reminded of it continuously. Our species evolved to eat and store fat for the long winter when food was scarce. We were not built for eating around the clock throughout the year. We were also not built for an environment in which stress is a constant undercurrent. Craving for food is fueled by stress. In our earliest human history, the energy from food was needed to react quickly and fight off a saber-toothed tiger. Either the tiger prevailed, or we did. But when stress is a constant and never resolved in such a clear-cut way, the brain's circuitry is thrown chronically off-kilter. As child psychiatrist Ned Hallowell writes in his book *Crazybusy*, we as a culture have grown accustomed to a lifestyle so fast-paced that we suffer from culturally-induced attention deficit hyperactivity disorder (ADHD) and continuously toxic levels of stress.

Although we label disordered eating an "epidemic", the problem comes not only from cues and substances in the environment to which we are passively exposed. Disordered eating comes from a complex interplay between our lifestyle choices, our history and, most importantly, our individual biochemistry. We can change how we eat and better understand emotional issues that may coexist with an eating problem. Most importantly, we can use science to find our way off the roller coaster. As the problem of disordered eating is fundamentally biological, so is the solution.

If your life involves a pattern of bingeing, shame, and restricted eating, this book will foster hope. You will learn the basic biochemistry behind food addiction and how your brain is caught in a cycle of pleasure and need. Then you can unleash the power of science to change your relationship with food.

Many of my colleagues who work with disordered eating believe they must be entrenched in one camp or another: they must treat their patients with medications *or* offer psychotherapy *or* recommend nutritional supplements. My approach does not suggest that there is ONE answer to binge eating. Instead, mine is a comprehensive approach that evolves from the field of integrative medicine. This, the New Hope model outlined in this book, integrates nutritional therapies along with medications, psychotherapy, and other lifestyle changes as needed. It is dysregulation in the brain that causes the appetite to run wild. Consequently, the New Hope model is designed to restore brain health. A return to brain health brings invites the realization of mental and emotional freedom as well as physical balance and well-being, ending a frantic and tortured roller-coaster ride.

This book will not arouse false hope about the next new diet. Instead, the New Hope will help you to stop feeling shame and to change your relationship with food. Following these guidelines, you will find your answers to appetite control and your path off the roller coaster.

PART I.
THE ROLLER-COASTER RIDE OF BINGE EATING AND FOOD ADDICTION

1
THE NEW HOPE: RESTORING CONTROL

The roller-coaster ride gets old. You've plunged through its jerks and twists a thousand times. You successfully resist cravings for several weeks. Then comes a momentary lapse in vigilance and, once again, eating spins out of control. The needle on the scale that you watched descend just days ago inches back up again. A critical inner voice berates you for your lack of willpower and plays in your head like a broken record. This scenario, an all-too-familiar roller-coaster ride, seems hopeless.

No matter how many times you have ridden this roller coaster, there is good reason to hope that this time you WILL get your appetite under control. You have failed in the past because you—with the help of the medical profession and the food environment of our culture—have misplaced the blame for your disordered eating. You may have explained your overeating as the result of a weak will or bad character. But the problem you struggle with is not a moral or character weakness; it is a biochemical one. Recognizing that cravings for food come from deep within our biochemistry and outside our conscious control should lead us to see disordered eating through a different lens. And just as we have misdiagnosed the problem of binge eating and overeating in the past, we have until now missed finding effective, permanent solutions.

But things have changed, and you can change, too. We now have a much more accurate understanding of the complicated, neurochemical process of appetite. We now know that food cravings are the manifestations of a genetically-based biochemical disorder that skews the body's natural signals of hunger and satiety (fullness).

As the problem we once attributed to laziness or lack of self-discipline is actually biochemical, so is the solution. That is the New Hope. In this book I will explain how we can adjust individual biochemistry to return appetite to normal levels. When biochemistry is adjusted, you can control your appetite without constant vigilance and self-restraint. You will actually lose interest in overeating!

Does this seem impossible to believe? The definition of hope is belief in things you cannot yet see, so I am asking you now to take hope based on my experience. As a psychiatrist in practice for more than twenty years, I have witnessed thousands of patients regain a normal relationship with food and appetite. It can happen to you, too.

First, a brief look at biochemistry will explain why cravings for food can be so intense. Palatable foods rich in sugar and fat stimulate the reward and pleasure centers of the brain. When you experience intense pleasure associated with sugar-laden foods, your brain produces a rush of dopamine in the reward pathway. This dopamine release creates the cycle of craving, followed by withdrawal, making you quickly crave food again. This craving is so strong for some of us that it overrides the brain's signals of fullness and satisfaction and the rational intention for self-care. Therefore, you keep eating even when you are not hungry. Although you eat more, food satisfies you less and less. This is the definition of *tolerance*, a hallmark condition of addiction.

According to the American Society of Addiction Medicine, addiction is a primary, chronic disease of brain reward, motivation, memory and related circuitry. Dysfunction in these circuits leads to characteristic biological, psychological, social, and spiritual manifestations. The individual hyper-focuses on pursuing reward and relief by ingesting more of the addictive substance. Eventually, life becomes an out-of-control rollercoaster ride. Food addiction is specifically defined as a chronic, relapsing problem that encompasses three phases: 1) binge intoxication, 2) withdrawal and 3) craving.

If you think "addiction" is too strong a word to apply to food, you might find experimental studies performed with rats to be very enlightening. Scientists often use rats in their research because rodent brains react to addictive substances in much the same way that human brains do. Studying rats has yielded an astonishing wealth of insight about appetite, particularly on the effects of rats' sugar consumption on levels of dopamine in pleasure centers of their brains. Chapter 6 in this book discusses the undeniable evidence from research of the addictive power of sugar. One of the strongest neurochemical commonalities between sugar binges and alcohol binges is their effects on dopamine. When hungry rats drink a sugar solution, dopamine is released in a region of their brain known as the nucleus accumbens. This triggers the motivation to consume more. More sugar provokes another surge of dopamine. After a month of daily sugar consumption, the rats' brains actually adapt in structure and function to increased dopamine levels. They have fewer *dopamine receptors* (specialized molecules on the exterior surfaces of brain cells that recognize and bind to dopamine) than they had before; consequently, they need more of the substance to produce the same sense of satisfaction. When they again have access to sugar, their consumption increases. Essentially, they learn to binge. Finally, when sugar water is introduced to their cages, they drink it all at once. In fact, they are drawn to sugar water even more urgently than to cocaine. Rats that consume sugar solutions develop all three phases of addiction: binge intoxication, withdrawal, and craving.

The effects of sugar on rats are mirrored in humans. Overeating blunts the dopamine reward response, encouraging overeating. When people eat large amounts of processed junk foods, which are purposely engineered to excite the dopamine system, the brain over time *down-regulates* (decreases the number of) its own dopamine receptors, and less dopamine is made available. This decrease leads to a yearning for reinforcement, which both weakens the ability to resist temptation and diminishes the satisfaction that can be obtained from food. A study conducted in 2011 revealed that women who gained significant amounts of weight over six months experienced a reduced dopamine response to highly palatable foods, which prompted them to eat more in order to stimulate dopamine production. Therein lies the vicious cycle of addiction!

Not everyone who eats sugar becomes addicted to it, just as not everyone who drinks alcohol becomes an alcoholic. During the last couple of decades, genetics researchers identified a gene marker for alcoholism that is associated with dopamine receptors in the brain. More recent investigation has concluded that most overeaters have the same genetic marker as alcoholics.

Palatable foods activate other neural systems besides dopamine. The opioids also play a major role in the reward circuit by stimulating opioid receptors in the brain. Not to be confused with opiates, a pharmacologic term for substances derived from the opium plant that are used to make drugs such as morphine, codeine, and heroin, *opioids* are molecules produced naturally by the body. The fact that the body produces opioid molecules may come as a surprise to many, as the word 'opioid' likely conjures darkly-tinged associations with illegal drug use. But it does: the human genome contains genes that code for opioid peptides (molecules made up of amino acids), opioid cell receptors are located throughout the central nervous system and digestive tract, and specialized, opioid-producing neurons are scattered throughout the body that together are known as the *endogenous opioid system*. The opioids these neurons create – beta-endorphins, met- and leu-enkephalins, and dynorphins – act as neurotransmitters and neuromodulators and cause a variety of effects such as pain relief, anxiety reduction, mood alterations, and reward-seeking behavior.

It is the last of these effects – reward-seeking – that that makes opioids so significant when it comes to perpetuating food addictions. Humans produce opioid peptides as a derivative of digesting excess sugar and fat. This cycle begins as the individual eats an excessive quantity of sugar or fat, then restricts intake, then binges again. The body produces increasing amounts of its own opioids which, we must remember, have the same chemical structure as the active ingredient in opiate drugs like morphine and heroin. Individuals experience a high, followed by withdrawal and craving, similar to what they would experience by ingesting an opiate drug.

The power of the biochemical effects of palatable food is even more striking when those effects are blocked. An important study investigated the effects of the medication naltrexone, a common opioid/opiate blocker, on disordered eating. The participants in the study were addicted to junk food; then, when they were given naltrexone, they simply lost interest in it. The results of this original study have since been replicated, revealing without a doubt that opioids were the culprits in fueling a yearning for food.

Also implicated in the addictive potential of food are morphine-like substances derived from dairy and wheat. *Casomorphins*, opioid peptides derived from the milk protein *casein*, are morphine analogs that have neuroactive properties, meaning they can modify the activities of nerves. As casein proteins are digested, they break apart to release casomorphins. The evolutionary purpose behind casomorphins is clear: mother's milk has a calming effect. But cheese, which is ten times more concentrated than milk, delivers a casomorphin payload in great excess of what the human body is chemically designed to handle. *Gliadorphins* are opiate peptides derived from the protein *gluten*, which is found in various cereal grains (primarily wheat, barley, rye, and oats). Like casomorphins, gliadorphins can react with opioid receptors in the brain, mimicking the effects of opiate drugs. Casomorphin and gliadorphin are food-derived molecules that are normal byproducts of digestion when they can be properly broken down to amino acids.

The casomorphins and gliadorphins are examples of the problematic interaction of food substances with individual biochemistry. Not everyone is susceptible to the addictive potential of opiates from these foods. The levels become elevated only when casein and gluten are partially digested and cross into the brain. If they are not broken down into amino acids and safely absorbed into the blood stream, the gliadorphin or casomorphin can cause addictive cravings for wheat or dairy products. Casomorphin and gliadorphin will be discussed in more detail in chapter 7.

Even though not everyone has the same degree of susceptibility to these peptides, everyone with a biochemistry that makes them vulnerable will likely develop craving symptoms. Three-fourths of the calories we consume as part of the Standard Western Diet come from dairy and wheat products. In fact, the Standard Western Diet, rich in processed foods laden with refined carbohydrates, saturated fats, and sugars, sets the stage for vulnerable individuals to become addicted to foods that are a part a daily routine. We have a bountiful universe of food options that have been engineered to deliver sugar and fat as cheaply as possible. Dr. David Kessler, former Commissioner of the FDA, considers salt an additional substance that tips the reward system of the brain to overwhelm rational choice. The trio of sugar, fat and salt, he contends, is mutually reinforcing. These are the foods that lead to chemical imbalances and trigger binges; after all, no one binges on broccoli. Our brains are ill equipped to manage these chemical imbalances. Over time, brain circuitry gone awry crystallizes as addiction.

The fascinating research into the effects of sugar on experimental rats provides clear evidence of the process and power of addiction to food. Fortunately, although the human brain can be held hostage to addiction, we also possess the ability to stand back, observe ourselves, and change. Following an individualized plan to stabilize biochemical imbalances with food can break the addictive cycle of bingeing and restore a trustworthy appetite.

Our ability to realize that we have misattributed the source of the problem and then to shift course and change is fundamental to the New Hope model. Overeating is a biologically-based disorder that requires biologically-based solutions. In this book, I will explain more about the types of foods that can trigger addiction. I will show you how to address nutritional deficiencies that may contribute to patterns of disordered and binge eating. I will also suggest lifestyle changes that will help you find your own way out of food addiction and disordered eating. You WILL get off the roller coaster.

Over many years, I have treated thousands of patients suffering from appetite disturbances. I have developed a science-based approach to binge eating. This is an integrative approach founded on the insights from current medical research combined with natural strategies. Because appetite disorders are caused by a combination of many factors, an integrative approach provides the best - and most lasting - solution. This multi-faceted approach offers real hope to the millions who struggle with binge eating and other eating disturbances.

Integrative medicine is a therapeutic approach to healing that treats the whole patient as an individual. It is based on biochemical individuality and on the understanding that the body, mind and spirit are interconnected. The goal is to restore balance in the body by adjusting and strengthening the factors, both internal and external, which allow the body to function optimally. Integrative medicine differs from conventional medicine, which views each body system as an isolated entity and the mind as separate from the body.

While integrative medicine leverages important tools that most physicians would never think of because they are outside the confines of the traditional discipline, it is also solidly based in scientific medicine. It begins with a scientific assessment to determine your nutritional needs—what nutrients are missing, in excess or out of proportion. This is coupled with an evaluation of any coexisting conditions that may contribute to your disordered eating.

It makes sense: before you can find a solution to a problem, you need to understand its exact contours. Fundamental to success is a comprehensive metabolic evaluation to uncover any physical or nutritional abnormalities that might be contributing to your appetite problems. The test results reveal your unique metabolic and nutritional profile, which will then become the foundation of your program.

Understanding the neurobiology of addiction and your own genetic make-up should help you stop blaming yourself! Recognizing that we are all influenced, but not determined, by our genes should help you see the importance of an individualized strategy for appetite control. Addressing the challenges of co-occurring conditions like depression and ADHD are part of tailoring a program for you.

Once you identify genetic, emotional and nutritional factors that may lead you to overeat, you can shift the blame for overeating from your character to your biochemistry, where it rightly belongs. From this foundation, you can treat disordered eating patterns, attacking problems at their source rather than simply—and temporarily—eradicating symptoms.

Just as there is rarely only one contributing factor to disordered eating, there is rarely one simple solution. The forces that fuel binge eating and food addiction are complex. Beware of books or speakers that promise One True Way to regaining control over appetite! I have found that once the nature of an individual's eating patterns has been carefully identified, recovery is most successful with a combination of three interventions: (1) nutritional supplementation, (2) medications if needed and (3) lifestyle changes. You can use one or all of these interventions, depending on how your body responds.

Nutritional Supplementation

When the body lacks certain nutrients, brain chemistry and even brain structure are affected. Nutritional deficiencies routinely cause physical and emotional problems that complicate the diagnosis and treatment of disordered eating. Nutritional deficiencies can trigger symptoms of disordered eating, delaying treatment and fostering the chronic cycle of relapse after periods of recovery.

There are several reasons why nutritional deficiencies are largely ignored by mental health treatment programs. Chief among them is the fact that most doctors lack nutritional knowledge, and while textbooks offer precise lists of symptoms caused by deficiencies of specific nutrients, the real-world relationships between nutrient deficiencies and symptoms are often not clear.

In the middle of the twentieth century, Roger Williams, PhD, formulated the concept of *biochemical individuality*, based on the idea that each person needs different levels of nutrients for optimal health and functioning and, accordingly, has a unique response to nutritional deficiencies. Evidence of the validity and legitimacy of this concept has been around for centuries. For instance, in the eighteenth century, sailors on long voyages sometimes developed scurvy, a disease caused by lack of vitamin C. A seafaring chaplain, Richard Walter, observed that the disease seemed to have as many different symptoms as people who suffered from it: "…for scarcely two persons have the same complaints and where there is found some conformity in symptoms, the order of their appearance has been totally different."

In my practice, I see tremendous individual variation in physical and psychological symptoms among people with the same nutritional deficiencies. Erratic eating, fasting, and purging can lead to nutritional deficiencies that are associated with both physical and psychological complications. For instance, a deficiency of essential fatty acids is correlated with depression, bipolar disorder, and ADHD. A lack of B vitamins and vitamin C contributes to depression and fatigue, and too little magnesium can result in anxiety, constipation, and insomnia. Chromium deficiency has been linked to depression and increased appetite. Taking the nutritional supplements your body needs to correct these problems can help regulate cravings and disordered eating.

In Chapter 8, you'll learn about laboratory testing to determine your individualized biochemical profile. Chapter 10 will help identify nutritional supplements helpful for appetite regulation and food cravings.

In addition to needing vitamin and mineral supplements, I have found that most of my patients who struggle with disordered eating also need supplementation with amino acids. *Amino acids* are the raw materials your body uses to produce the neurotransmitters and neuropeptides responsible for controlling appetite. Low levels of neurotransmitters can result in depression, anxiety, sugar and carbohydrate cravings, overeating, and bingeing. Amino acid supplementation can normalize both appetite and mood. Amino acid supplements will not simply mask the symptoms of eating disturbances but will instead target – and eliminate – the root causes of such symptoms.

In Chapter 9, you'll learn about amino acids that can stop cravings and binge eating—including 5-HTP, phenylalanine, and tyrosine—and amino acid blends that I have found most effective in treating disordered eating. Many patients have found that nutritional supplements, in combination with amino acids, are enough to transform their relationship with food.

Medications

Only one medication is currently approved by the United States Food and Drug Administration (FDA) for a type of disordered eating: fluoxetine (Prozac) for treating bulimia. Other problems related to eating, including anorexia, obsessive dieting, binge eating, and compulsive overeating, have no approved pharmaceutical treatment. Research has provided clear evidence that individual medications for patients with appetite disturbances have limited value. However, medication combinations can provide tremendous biological relief from out-of-control eating behaviors and halt the roller-coaster ride.

While there is no one magic pill, medication is also not the enemy! Sometimes a medication or combination of medications is a necessary augmentation to the nutritional treatments for appetite disturbances. Chapter 11 describes the medications I have found most helpful, especially selective serotonin reuptake inhibitors (SSRIs), Topamax, Zonisamide, and Naltrexone. Recent research has shown that medications indicated for the treatment of coexisting psychiatric problems, such as depression and ADHD, can have tremendous benefit for binge eating as well.

Lifestyle Changes

We are routinely bombarded with fad diets that promise 'magic bullet' methods to achieve weight loss and longevity. The problem is that what constitutes a 'perfect' diet changes with each new celebrity book that rolls off the press. Most of you are already aware of what a healthy diet looks like. The problem isn't not knowing what to do, but rather in doing, implementing, and living what you know. The final intervention for appetite control is lifestyle changes. These changes include avoiding foods that trigger your particular biochemical sensitivities and eating foods that normalize appetite and metabolism. Chapters 12 and 13 describe the importance of avoiding food additives, including high fructose corn syrup (HFCS) and monosodium glutamate (MSG). High fructose corn syrup throws the brain's reward system out of kilter, setting in motion a process that can lead to addiction. The glutamate in MSG stimulates insulin production, leading to overeating. Chapter 14, *Controlling Appetite with an UN-Diet*, explains how eating under stressful circumstances can hinder optimal digestion. Eating regular meals and snacks in a relaxing environment will set the stage for you to control your appetite while living diet-free.

Another important lifestyle change you can make is to recognize that you are not alone and to seek support from others. Participating in individual therapy, group therapy, or Twelve- Step programs can make the difference in achieving long-term relief from disordered eating and finding enjoyable human connections along the way. Psychotherapy can help you explore emotions that may have fueled disordered evening. Cognitive-behavioral therapy (CBT), which trains the individual to recognize faulty patterns of thinking and replace unhealthy thoughts with healthier ones, has been shown to be especially effective in people struggling to regain control over appetite. Group therapy and mindfulness offer perspective to help solve the problems that keep disordered eating patterns in play. Recent research suggests that participation in a Twelve-Step program not only helps participants find a sense of belonging with others who have similar struggles, but that the program's philosophy of shifting the problem away from a defect in will power and reframing one's personal story also activates the dopamine system in ways that are even visible on brain scans. A religious orientation is not a prerequisite to participating in a Twelve-Step program.

Chapter 15 tells you more about types of therapy that might help you. Finally, make sure you balance movement and rest. Movement and rest are the yin and yang of health. Exercise is critical for all of us. Strenuous aerobic exercise, including jogging, tennis, basketball, skating, cycling, etc., suppresses the appetite during the exercise session and at least for a brief time afterward. This is because aerobic exercise alters certain hormone levels. Specifically, it decreases levels of the hormone ghrelin, which fuels hunger, while increasing the appetite-quelling hormone PYY. In addition, aerobic exercise eases anxiety and stress, other triggers of uncontrolled eating. Sleep is known to be a factor in helping to control appetite, as sleep stimulates the production of leptin, which curbs appetite. Conversely, loss of sleep interferes with the body's ability to metabolize carbohydrates and contributes to the storage of fat throughout the body.

In Chapter 16, you'll read about exercise and sleep and how they can help you regulate your body's appetite controls.

I have watched many people joyfully reclaim control over their appetite and enjoy all the health benefits that come from ending a pattern of disordered eating. This integrative approach, which treats an appetite gone wild as the complex problem it is, offers New Hope to the millions who struggle day after day, year after year, to keep their eating under control. The approach I have outlined is not new; what *is* new is the *combination of interventions* brought together in an integrative program to solve a complicated, multi-faceted problem.

Following the New Hope model, you can get off the roller coaster and approach food with pleasure unclouded by guilt and shame. This has been your goal. Even if you have lost hope and this sense of enjoyment for years or even decades, it is yours to reclaim. The New Hope can become your new reality.

Summary

Millions of people struggle with appetite control, binge eating, and other eating disturbances. Tormented by food cravings, those who suffer from chronic overeating are left on an anguishing roller-coaster ride of difficult emotions, social challenges, and destructive physical consequences. Many have found the flashy diets and popular weight loss programs advertised in the media to be ineffective, only increasing their feelings of guilt, isolation, and utter hopelessness.

Traditional treatment approaches for appetite problems have failed because our culture and beliefs about food have prevented us from recognizing that biochemical imbalances are the foundation of disordered eating. Food addictions cannot be resolved by willpower alone. It is only by understanding the complex physiological phenomenon of appetite and the genetic, emotional, and nutritional factors controlling it that a solution is possible.

Combining the latest in medical research with over thirty years of clinical psychiatric experience, the following chapters offer an integrative solution for individuals trapped in destructive patterns of disordered eating. Using a holistic model, this book describes the combination of metabolic testing, nutritional supplementation, medications, and lifestyle changes needed to rebalance biochemistry and make the rediscovery of a a healthy relationship with food possible. For many, this book will be the New Hope they have been waiting for.

Key Points

- Chronic overeating can be a tormenting roller-coaster ride of cravings, restraint, guilt, isolation and hopelessness.
- Many treatment approaches are ineffective because they do not recognize that appetite disturbance is actually a deep biochemical phenomenon that cannot be resolved by effort and willpower alone.
- This book explains how to treat disordered eating by healing the whole person and recognizing that complex genetic, emotional and nutritional factors all influence food behaviors.
- Genetic and biochemical factors powerfully influence our individual responses to food, making certain items desirable and highly addictive.
- Palatable foods rich in sugar, fat and salt stimulate the rewards centers in the brain, triggering a rush of dopamine that trips the cycle of craving.
- Some of the most popular foods in the Standard American Diet, such as wheat and dairy, contain morphine-like compounds that can be overwhelmingly habit-forming in sensitive individuals.
- Research has shown that the additives in many processed foods act like opioids in the body, creating food obsessions and skewing natural signals of hunger and satiety.

- Erratic eating habits, fasting and purging create metabolic disturbances and nutrient deficiencies that result in complicating physical and emotional symptoms.
- Similar to other types of chemical dependency, addictions to food involve three chronically relapsing phases: binge intoxication, withdrawal and craving.
- The New Hope model explained in this book describes an integrative approach for treating food addiction and binge eating disorder, which draws on the neurobiology of addiction as a scientific foundation.

2
ADDICTED TO FOOD:
MY DOPAMINE MADE ME DO IT

Addiction is a powerful word. It unleashes feelings of helplessness, anxiety, and chaos. For many of us, the word evokes the image of a particular person. We may have watched someone for whom a substance—alcohol or another drug—became so important that everything else faded into insignificance. Acquiring the drugs or alcohol became an all-consuming goal regardless of the consequences.

The behavior of an addict baffles many. We all know stories of people whose rational thinking and ability to cope were held hostage by drug addiction. What does this have to do with food? The answer is that people can be addicted to food, too. Of course, unlike alcohol or cocaine, food is not a drug that people can elect to do without; nevertheless, certain foods and patterns of disordered eating can set an addictive process in motion. Food addiction, like addiction to alcohol or another drug, hijacks the brain. People don't rationally decide to eat everything in the refrigerator late at night or secretly make themselves vomit. Instead, they eat or eat and purge in an urgent, disordered way and against their better judgment. What classifies their behavior as an addiction is not the substance itself, but the relationship between the substance—in this case, food—and their brains.

Perhaps identifying food as an addictive substance does not surprise you. The subject of food addiction has reached the mass media, which features everything from scientific bulletins to best-sellers about celebrities acknowledging their own secret struggles with food. Dr. Pamela Peeke, in *The Hunger Fix*, offers fitness suggestions and customized meal plans to help break dependence on the sugary, salty high-fat foods most likely to trigger addiction. Mika Brzezinski, cohost of MSNBC's *Morning Joe*, released her personal story in *Obsessed: America's Food Addiction and My Own*. After verbal jousts for years with her cohost Joe Scarborough, who talked up McDonald's burgers while she extolled the virtues of the "healthy" food that kept her skinny, she acknowledged in *Obsessed* her years of secret binge eating and purging. Now out from under secrecy and unhealthy food rituals, she expresses both relief and humility as to the power of food addiction: "It's like alcoholism. Every day is a new day. I take one day at a time."

Food addiction is a daunting opponent because it occurs deep in the brain; it is a biochemical process. You may struggle with the false hope that next time you will eat differently. But if you are rigorously honest with yourself, you know what will really happen next time. As long as you try to avoid recognizing how intractable this pattern is, you use up energy that could be channeled toward solving the problem. There are millions of people in this country who have acknowledged an addiction and who are now recovering successfully from it.

Comparing food addiction and alcohol addiction yields two very important realizations. One, we have long known that alcohol addiction is the result of biochemical processes gone haywire; it is a disease. If addiction to food follows the same pathway, then eating out of control and succumbing yet again to the temptation to binge is the result of a biochemical process and not a deficiency of willpower. Addiction to food is not your fault! This book will describe the recent scientific research that demonstrates the biochemical underpinnings of food addiction.

Second, and just as important, there *is* something you can do about it! I'm not talking about the inner monologues of shame with which you beat yourself up after overeating, or unrealistic hope in the promise of yet another new diet plan that you'll start tomorrow. While these "solutions" are destined to be ineffectual, there is a way to take control of your relationship with food. You can discover how your unique biochemistry, triggered by foods that you eat, sets up the powerful cycle of addiction. Addiction is a formidable force, but by understanding the process, you can break free.

To recognize parallel patterns in addictions to drugs and to food, let's look first at psychiatry's usual method of determining if a person is dependent upon alcohol or another drug. The *Diagnostic and Statistical Manual of Mental Disorders*, or the *DSM*, is the standard reference that psychiatrists around the world use to diagnose and categorize mental and emotional disorders. The *DSM* determines whether to classify a person as dependent on a substance by asking questions about tolerance, withdrawal, difficulty controlling use, desire to cut down, and specific negative consequences. If his or her answer is "yes" to three or more of the following questions - which I have revised to focus specifically on food - a person is dependent.

1. **Tolerance:** Has your use of *food* increased over time?
2. **Withdrawal:** When you stop *eating*, have you ever experienced physical or emotional withdrawal? Have you had any of the following symptoms: irritability, anxiety, shakes, sweats, nausea or vomiting?
3. **Difficulty controlling your use:** Do you sometimes *eat* more or for a longer time than you would like? Do you sometimes *eat* to *numb yourself*? Do you stop after a few *bites* usually, or does one *binge/purge* lead to more *binge/purge episodes*?
4. **Negative consequences:** Have you continued a *pattern of disordered eating* even though there have been negative consequences to your mood, self-esteem, health, job or family?
5. **Neglecting or postponing activities:** Have you ever put off or reduced social, recreational, work or household activities because of your *eating patterns or your weight*?
6. **Spending significant time or emotional energy:** Have you spent a significant amount of time obtaining, using, concealing, planning or recovering from your *eating patterns*? Have you spent a lot of time thinking about *eating*? Have you ever concealed or minimized your *eating habits*? Have you ever thought of schemes to avoid getting caught?

7. **Desire to cut down:** Have you sometimes thought about cutting down or controlling your *eating*? Have you ever made unsuccessful attempts to cut down or control your *eating patterns*?

You may find that the answer "yes" rings true to many of these questions about your own relationship with food. Eating, thoughts about eating, regrets about eating, and planning to eat may organize your life. Food may have assumed an importance and urgency far beyond what you ever intended. This is what an addiction looks like.

New research about disordered eating led the developers of the *DSM-V*, the newest version of the psychiatric manual published in May 2013, to include binge eating disorder for the first time as a classifiable disease. This establishment of formal, diagnostic criteria makes it possible for people with binge eating disorder to receive professional treatment with health insurance coverage. It also raises awareness about the seriousness of disordered eating as a medical illness.

Addiction is a chronic, relapsing disorder that encompasses three distinct phases: a binge intoxication phase; a withdrawal phase accompanied by negative emotions as the drug's effects diminish; and a preoccupation and anticipation phase that leads to using more of the addictive substance. The substance actually changes the chemistry of the brain, which then prompts an intensified need for it. Recent scientific research shows clearly why some people become addicted to food. Neural correlates, or processes in the brain, underlie these behavioral patterns that contribute to all addictive behaviors.

To appreciate the process that goes haywire in the addicted person, it helps to understand the structure of the brain. The *cortex* is the part of the brain in which conscious thought occurs and is the part of the brain that makes us distinctively human. The cortex is also called the "new brain" because, from an evolutionary point of view, it appears in more highly evolved species such as lower primates and humans. The cortex houses the superior mental faculties—memory, learning, and judgment. It is, in fact, the part on which all conscious thought is based.

Despite its amazing properties, however, the human cortex is baffled by addiction. To see why, we must look at other parts of the brain, regions that control the reward circuit and are the seat of our most basic drives: hunger, thirst, the fight-or-flight reaction, sex, and pain regulation. These include the amygdala, the insula, and the striatum. Although the cortex may appear to be running the show, the reward circuit wields deceptive power.

From the perspective of addiction, the reward circuit is where the action is. For treatment to be effective, the brain must be educated about the errors in circuitry by which it has been baffled. You can't think your way out of addiction. The role of the reward circuit shows why even the most sophisticated analytical thinking cannot provide the basis for change. For a long time, a tragic error in treatment for addiction was the mistaken belief that if the addict could develop enough insight into his problems and come to feel better about himself through psychotherapy, he could stop his addictive behavior. Sadly, the relapse histories of countless patients proved this to be a critical error. To the addict, no amount of insight about underlying causes is enough to overcome the biologic craving for chemical relief.

Changes in the wiring of the reward circuit that result from drug addiction are not just metaphorical; they are actual alterations to the physical structure of the brain, and visible using brain imaging technologies like positron emission tomography (PET) scans. On PET scans performed while abstinent addicts are watching a videotape of cues associated with drinking or injecting drugs, the amygdala, an almond-shaped structure buried in the temporal lobe of the brain, lights up on the screen. This means that the mere anticipation of drug use—filling a syringe, even watching a commercial advertising alcohol on television—stimulates chemical changes in the brain before the drug itself is even ingested!

More recent research shows exactly the same effect when someone who struggles with disordered eating is presented with food cues. A picture of a juicy cheeseburger flashes on the screen and the person's amygdala lights up at the mere thought of tasting it, indicating a surge of activity in regions of the brain that govern cravings. In other words, actually eating or even tasting food isn't necessary to chemically prime the reward circuit to induce a physical reaction. The thought itself sets in motion the frightening neurochemical nightmare we call addiction.

Addictive substances, including foods, stimulate the release of dopamine, which is the major neurotransmitter in the brain's reward circuit. It is the release of dopamine that induces feelings of well-being or euphoria. As a person ingests more food to re-experience pleasure, the body develops tolerance. Whereas the short-term use of drugs or food increases dopamine levels, chronic use decreases dopamine, as well as the body's ability to produce it. Because the brain's natural mechanism for dopamine release is stalled, ever-larger fixes are needed to attain more-rapidly-diminishing effects. A blunted sense of reward then causes people to overeat in compensation. The resulting depletion of dopamine results in craving. Dr. Steven Hyman, former director of the National Institute of Mental Health, likens addictive substances to Trojan horses. In masquerade, they fool the brain into releasing dopamine, but as they wreak havoc with the brain's natural mechanism of regulating pleasure, the apparent gift becomes an agent of betrayal.

A research study published in the prestigious medical journal *The Lancet* found that overweight patients had significantly fewer dopamine receptors in their brains than normal-weight individuals. And as body weight increased in the overweight group, the number of dopamine receptors declined still more. This means that the brains of overweight patients had less dopamine available for use, even if normal amounts were produced, making them less sensitive to subtle dopamine rewards. This condition has been called *reward deficiency syndrome*. These patients were also more likely to indulge in other behaviors to find a sense of pleasure and release—like abuse of alcohol and other drugs.

In addition to experiencing less sense of reward from dopamine, people who are at risk for being overweight may have brains that are programmed to overeat fattening foods. In one study, when normal-weight women were shown pictures of high-calorie foods, activity in one decision-making part of the brain increased significantly. But in overweight women, the same pictures stimulated activity in *eleven* areas of the brain, including several parts of the limbic system, which plays an important role in reward and motivational processing.

An overactive limbic system may be one reason that overweight people have low levels of dopamine. When the limbic system is activated for long periods of time, the brain's ability to start and stop dopamine production is compromised, slowing the release of this important neurotransmitter. Eating more is required to continue to stimulate dopamine release. In addition, a hyperactive limbic system causes the release of increased amounts of a substance called deltaFosB, which motivates the search for more palatable foods. It may be that the limbic systems of people who are prone to weight problems may be hyper-responsive to both food cues and food rewards, driving the urge to overeat. This pattern closely replicates limbic system activity in people addicted to drugs.

The reward circuit in the brain plays a critical role in the maintenance of the body's equilibrium, health, and vitality by sending appropriate signals that "turn on" and "turn off" the urge to eat. When it doesn't function properly or becomes skewed by exposure to drugs of abuse or prolonged overeating, the reward circuit can fuel unhealthy drug use or eating behaviors.

In 2009, the journal *Addiction* published a paper by researchers at the Food Addiction Institute exploring the connection between physical cravings and food addiction. The authors call on public health professionals to design programs that treat food addiction based on proven models for treating other forms of substance abuse. Scientists point out that there is now more empirical evidence for physical craving as a component of food addiction than there was for physical craving as a manifestation of alcoholism when it was first defined as a substance abuse disorder. Yet when someone struggles with alcoholism, medical treatment and detox programs are available. Twelve-Step support groups meet in cities and towns throughout the country. These programs are based on the understanding that recovery is a complex process that takes time and group support. People who struggle with disordered eating, however, are often alone, have few affordable treatment options, and are less likely to find a group tailored to their specific needs.

Among the most destructive cultural attitudes toward addiction of any kind in our society is the notion that the addicted person is morally weak and lacks self-discipline. When internalized, this attitude interferes with an individual's realization that he has a disease and with his understanding of the insidious biochemical processes that trigger the addiction process.

Another destructive attitude is that relapse is a predictor of failure. In fact, many addiction specialists contend that the number of times a person has tried to take control of an addictive pattern such as alcoholism or addiction to food is a strong and positive predictor of success.

Many of you who struggle with disordered eating cope with all the elements of addiction: bingeing, withdrawal, and craving. Gradually, you seem motivated less by seeking the sense of reward from food than by avoiding the negative emotional state that results from withdrawal. Over and over again, the forces that drive you to eat win out over willpower, logic, and common sense. For many of the thousands of patients I have treated, binge eating, overeating, and obesity often result from neurochemical changes in the brain that mimic addiction. You feel like you've been on a never-ending roller-coaster ride and you cannot get off. Recent research underscores the validity of this description, as well as the tormented struggles I hear daily from men and women who have a constant fear of food, never-ending shame, and low self-esteem. The New Hope model explained in this book will help you break an addictive pattern to food and get off the roller coaster for good.

Summary

Over time, appetite dysregulation and disrupted eating patterns lead to an addictive process wherein the brain becomes chemically dependent on certain foods. Like addictions to alcohol and other drugs, an addiction to food creates biochemical changes that hijack the body's reward circuit. A pattern of chronic overeating alters the function of various centers in the brain, including the cortex, amygdala, and limbic system, and creates imbalances of dopamine, the "feel-good" neurotransmitter. Consequently, deep physical cravings become so strong that they are impossible to control simply by stubborn resolve or thought alone. Ruminations about food, regrets around meals, and emotional connections to foods become constant and burdensome, fueling a chronic and relapsing addiction that mimics addictions to other substances. However, with insight into your unique biochemistry, you can bring the disrupted pathways in the body back into equilibrium, breaking the cycle of addiction and restoring a trustworthy appetite.

If you believe that your appetite is out of control, the solution might begin with understanding that the underlying triggers might exist within the foods you crave. Part II will explore in-depth some of the components of food that drive addiction.

Key Points

- Certain foods and a pattern of disordered eating can create addictive processes.
- Constant thoughts about eating, regrets about eating, emotional ties to eating, an increase in food intake, and changes in social eating behaviors are all signs of food addiction.
- Like addictions to alcohol or another drug, food addiction causes deep biochemical changes in the brain that make it impossible to overcome with willpower alone.
- Disordered eating patterns disrupt the reward circuits of the brain—the pathway that keeps the body in equilibrium by turning the urge to eat "on" or "off."
- Prolonged overeating changes the function of the cortex, amygdala, and limbic system, and skews the release of dopamine, the "feel-good" neurotransmitter. These biochemical alterations shift the way we think about, feel about, and crave food.

3
THE APPETITE GONE WILD: MANY FORMS OF DISORDERED EATING

Although you might have thought appetite can be conquered through willpower and discipline, science is now revealing that it is not so simple.

It's not easy to change a pattern of disordered eating. Disordered eating results from complex interactions between genetics, hormones, vitamins, minerals, amino acids, stress, and personal habits. Moreover, the processes in the brain that perpetuate disordered eating lie outside our conscious control. We are frustrated because we fail at solving an eating problem with willpower. Willpower exists at the surface levels of the conscious mind, the tip of the iceberg. The powerful processes that keep the appetite running wild are in the vast part of the iceberg below the waterline.

At the deeper level, chemicals in the brain become wired to produce a powerful rush of pleasure in response to food or even the thought of it. In Chapter 2, I introduced the science of appetite and food addiction. Consuming sufficient quantities of food for energy metabolism is essential for the survival of all species in the animal kingdom. However, mammalian brains have evolved several interrelated neural and biochemical systems that drive feeding behaviors. The most potent driver of feeding behavior is its rewarding nature. We are no longer eating just to survive; we are seeking the feeling of happiness that is associated with eating certain foods.

An appetite gone wild can have many possible surface manifestations. Disturbances in appetite include excessive restriction of food, bingeing, bingeing and purging, night eating, and compulsive overeating.

These disturbances exist on a spectrum of severity, and range from mildly compulsive dieting to anorexia, from bingeing to binge eating disorder, and from occasional bingeing and purging to bulimia. Although rigidly-controlled dieting and chronic overeating may look like totally opposite behaviors, they have similar origins. To make the situation more complicated, appetite disorders may morph from one into another. A compulsive dieter may become a binge eater. As you can see, a great deal of fluidity exists among appetite disorders in both manifestation and severity.

What do these disturbances have in common? The chemicals in the brain intended to signal hunger and fullness, or satiety, have gone awry. Somehow, the physiological processes that control food intake have become so garbled that the body's natural signals can no longer be trusted.

It wasn't always that way. We are all born with instincts that tell us when to eat and when to stop. Even an infant "knows" these things, thanks to clear signals of hunger and fullness. A baby's stomach growls and she cries for food; when her stomach feels comfortably full, she pushes the food source away and doesn't care about eating until the hunger pangs return.

And for many adults these signals continue to work effectively. A person with a normal, healthy appetite will eat when she is hungry. She will neither eat beyond a comfortable state of fullness nor require heroic efforts to resist a persistent desire for more. After eating, she will simply forget about food until chemicals in the brain signal hunger again.

In some people, the inborn signals for hunger and satiety are out of kilter. What is indicative of an appetite has gone awry is not a person's size or weight; the key indicator is rather the degree of preoccupation with appetite and with satisfying or denying appetite. For instance, a compulsive dieter may be thin, but obsessed by measuring out portions of food and getting down to smaller and smaller clothing sizes. Appetite has taken on tremendous importance in her life; it has become her enemy. It has the power to make her gain weight, thereby flooding her with a sense of shame. If she can just wrestle her appetite to the ground and keep it there, the compulsive dieter believes she will finally be free to live a happy, peaceful life.

Of course, this never happens, as the wild and unfed appetite lies in wait for the inevitable slip in her vigilance and control. And even if the compulsive dieter is successful for a long time in keeping her appetite in a stranglehold, physical, mental and emotional problems take their toll. When the body is deprived of enough food, it works hard to conserve the small amount of energy it takes in. Metabolism slows, causing calories to burn at a lower rate. Heart rate and blood pressure drop, decreasing blood circulation. In women, menstrual periods can disappear, since a certain body fat level is essential to produce enough estrogen to keep the cycle going. Low estrogen in turn leads to decreased bone density, which may progress to osteoporosis. As food and nutrient deprivation continues, more severe physical problems develop: anemia, electrolyte imbalances, a decline in immune system function, heart arrhythmias, heart failure, kidney failure, and even death.

A person deprived of nutrients also begins to exhibit a wide range of emotional symptoms. The compulsive dieter is likely to become depressed. Eating behaviors become so strange—ritualistic patterns, cutting everything into micro bites, counting chews, hoarding food—that the person who lives this way becomes more and more isolated, trying to hide her elaborate behaviors involving food and its restriction. In short, her constant efforts to control her appetite take over her life.

At the opposite end of the spectrum of disordered eating is the person who eats far more than his body needs or can use. He responds to food cues by eating. This person is especially susceptible to the food stimuli everywhere in our culture. Passing a fast-food restaurant, going to the movies, seeing a billboard featuring a tasty cheeseburger, even thinking of a favorite food in the absence of an external cue triggers a bout of eating.

While our prehistoric ancestors benefited from eating as much as possible during times of plenty in order to be prepared for shortages that could lurk right around the corner, the biological mechanisms that protect our capacity to outlast famine not only are unnecessary in most parts of the modern world, they are also harmful. Today we are still wired to live in a food environment of scarcity and restriction, even as food is everywhere around us.

As you well know, chronic overeating leads to a host of physical, mental and emotional problems. An appetite out of control eventually leads to weight gain, causing shame and depression. More food, especially comfort foods that are soft and high in calories, are sought to soothe the neurochemical chaos induced by chronic overeating.

The Biology of the Binge

A particularly dangerous form of overeating is binge eating, which involves taking in excessive amounts of food over a short period in order to avoid bad feelings and to "normalize" mood. Binge eaters typically eat palatable foods and beverages that are high in sugar and fat. This food is not consumed in service of metabolic need; instead, it activates the reward pathways in the brain. As many as twenty thousand calories can be consumed in a single binge.

A binge eater usually begins with just a bite of a "forbidden" food. After experiencing that taste of chocolate cake, the binge eater suddenly throws all restraint to the wind and eats uncontrollably—in this case, the entire cake. The thought process is: "I've blown it. I might as well eat everything I want because I've already ruined my diet."

During a binge, the person eats rapidly, barely chewing. Agitated, anxious, and guilty, she is aware of what she is doing and is disgusted by it but feels powerless to stop. Once she is uncomfortably full and the binge is over, she feels remorseful, depressed, and angry at herself. It's not unusual for a person so beaten down by self-reproach to begin another binge in an hour or two. Because this process is surrounded with shame, binge eating is done mostly in secret.

A severe form of bingeing, binge eating disorder (BED), is defined as bingeing that occurs on average at least two days a week for a minimum of six months. The new *Diagnostic and Statistical Manual V*, published in May 2013, classifies binge eating disorder for the first time as a recognized mental disorder with predictable features. Binge eating disorder is the most common of all eating disorders and is correlated with the growing incidence of obesity. Yet there is little research devoted to this illness, and no approved medication to treat it.

In addition to causing chronic physical problems, bingeing leads to emotional distress. People who binge are typically mired in guilt, shame, and self-loathing, all of which increase depression and anxiety. Food, eating, and the time-consuming rituals of binge eating and its aftermath gradually overtake the place of family, friends, work, and hobbies in the binge eater's life, diminishing pleasure, happiness, and intimacy while increasing alienation, secrecy, and loneliness.

Night eating and a cycle of bingeing and purging are variations of binge eating, different manifestations of an appetite gone wild. Although night eaters have little appetite in the morning, appetite increases early in the afternoon and ramps up toward dinnertime. After dinner, the appetite becomes voracious and persistent. Sometimes food cravings are strong enough to wake people in the middle of the night. In patients who struggle with night eating, I often see depression, anxiety, and sleep problems.

The person who binges and purges tries desperately to control a wild appetite. To compensate for the overwhelming number of calories consumed during binges, many such individuals turn to self-induced vomiting, excessive exercise, or use of laxatives or diuretics.

The self-image of the person who binges and purges, like that of the compulsive dieter, is dependent upon the maintenance of a certain weight or shape. Even as a measure of restricting calories, purging is ineffective. Self-induced vomiting may rid the body of the calories most recently consumed, but some food will have made it into the small intestine where it is "safe" from being orally expelled. Laxatives and enemas target the large intestine or the colon, but by the time the digestive contents reach these areas, most calories have already been extracted. Diuretics don't affect food intake or fat stores; they just rid the body of water and electrolytes and only temporarily lower the number on the scale.

Moreover, the bingeing-purging cycle is dangerous. Purging can lead to an irritated or even ruptured esophagus. Tooth enamel is eroded by continual exposure to stomach acid, increasing the likelihood of cavities and making the teeth look ragged. Other problems include electrolyte imbalance, dehydration, vitamin and mineral deficiencies, chronic kidney problems, swollen parotid glands ("chipmunk cheeks"), and knuckle abrasions. Drugs used to induce vomiting may lead to heart problems or even heart failure. Diuretics and laxatives used over long periods can cause serious gastrointestinal problems.

The binge-purge cycles may cause or exacerbate symptoms of depression, anxiety, irritability, fatigue, shame, and guilt, intensifying the low self-esteem and out-of-control feelings that are the root of many appetite disturbances. The all-encompassing focus on an out-of-control appetite interferes with a person's ability to handle responsibilities, to grow, to learn, and to be happy.

The basis of an appetite gone wild is biochemical imbalance. After an evaluation of the underlying factors that may throw your appetite out of control, the New Hope model will make it possible for you to regain a normal appetite. Nutritional supplementation, medications if needed, and changes in your lifestyle replace the chaos of an abnormal appetite with a harmonious relationship with food. This can happen to you!

Summary

Disordered eating is a complex problem that can arise due to many interlinking factors, including genetics, hormones, nutrients, amino acids, stress, and personal habits. Although we are all born with instincts that help us decide when to eat and when to stop, in some people these innate signals are not functioning properly. The result is an appetite gone wild: eating patterns become sporadic, and uncontrollable chemical cravings for food develop. Thoughts and feelings about food take over, and an addictive process results, leading to an intense preoccupation with satisfying or conquering an unpredictable appetite.

Attempting to control these urges, people develop destructive eating patterns that include such damaging behaviors as bingeing, purging, and compulsive dieting. These behaviors exist along a spectrum of severity, and may range from bingeing to binge eating disorder, bingeing and purging to bulimia, and frequent dieting to anorexia. All, in turn, only strengthen the addiction to food, taking over the reward circuits of the brain and causing deep biological imbalances. With the wide variety of damaging physical, mental, and emotional symptoms that are associated with disordered eating, the struggle is impossible to overcome with willpower alone. However, when you follow a personalized treatment program that targets specific imbalances, your appetite will normalize, and harmony can be restored in the body.

Key Points

- Disordered eating is caused by many factors, including genetics, hormones, synthetic chemicals, vitamins, minerals, amino acids, stress, and personal habits.
- We are all born with instincts that tell us when to eat and when to stop. In some people these inborn signals are not functioning properly, and their eating patterns become destructive.
- There is a spectrum of disordered eating, ranging from mildly compulsive dieting to anorexia, from bingeing to binge eating disorder, and from bingeing and purging to bulimia.
- Bingeing, purging, and compulsive dieting create a wide range of dangerous physical, mental, and emotional problems.
- At the root of all types of disordered eating is a process that involves a preoccupation with appetite and how to conquer or satisfy it.
- By restoring balance to the body with a personalized treatment plan, appetite signals can be normalized and health can be restored.

4
YOU ARE EXTRAORDINARY: THE GENETICS OF APPETITE AND WEIGHT CONTROL

This chapter is about you.

You are unique; there is no reality to "ordinary" or "normal." In 1976, Roger J. Williams, Ph.D., who I mentioned in Chapter 1, published a book titled *You Are Extraordinary*. In this simple-to-read paperback, Dr. Williams describes his concept of biochemical individuality. He contends that every individual is different not only in personality and appearance, but also in biochemical uniqueness, a concept which extends to anatomy, the metabolism of vitamins and minerals, and the way the body detoxifies drugs and chemicals.

In the next chapters, I want to explore the genetics of appetite and weight management and discuss how a genetic vulnerability to many psychiatric conditions—including anxiety, depression, and ADHD—might contribute to your struggles with disordered eating.

Genetics

Many of you who struggle with disordered eating might believe you are a victim of fate. "It's in my genes. My mother, my sister and my grandmother all struggle with appetite and weight problems. I don't have a chance."

Genes are the body's blueprints, detailed instructions that create both body and mind. They determine the form and function of each cell in the body and therefore make you who you are. They are passed on from one generation to the next, but in each new birth they are combined in a unique way.

Thanks to individual genetic makeup, each person is anatomically and biochemically unique, with his or her own way of responding to the environment. This uniqueness frames the way that each of us perceives and interacts with the world. For instance, when a family sits down to enjoy dinner, each member actually tastes a different dinner because of the unique distribution of taste receptors in the tongue.

Taste receptors can have a big impact on overeating, bingeing, or not eating enough. A study funded by the National Institute on Deafness and Other Communication Disorders (NIDCD) has shown that small variations in our genetic code can raise or lower our sensitivity to sweet tastes. This can also explain why some people are especially vulnerable to addiction to sweets. Taste receptors are overloaded with different flavors during every meal, and if your diet is unhealthy, then taste receptors adapt to enjoying those foods, thereby making spinach and kale taste unappealing.

The differences in how we perceive taste are due to our genetics. Those with a sense of taste far more intense than that of the general population are called "supertasters." Supertasters have an aversion to bitter tastes, and studies have shown that supertasters also have a heightened risk of developing an affinity for eating salty foods, which masks bitterness.

Undoubtedly, there is a relationship between genetics and a predisposition for food addiction. A survey of Overeaters Anonymous members conducted in the early 1990s found that a high percentage of overeaters or food addicts had at least one blood relative also addicted to food or alcohol.

But this and other research raises the age-old question of nature versus nurture. Do these striking correlations run in families because the trait of susceptibility to addiction is passed on genetically? Or is it transmitted in habits and attitudes through patterns of parenting?

Scientific research has demonstrated that differences in DNA predispose individuals to alcohol dependence. Now science has linked genes with food addiction as well. Recently, researchers at the UCLA College of Medicine tested a sample of overweight subjects who exhibited a pattern of bingeing on carbohydrates. They found these subjects had exactly the same genetic aberration that had been established as a genetic marker for chemical dependency on alcohol.

But genetics is not destiny. You may have inherited genes that can predispose you to become addicted to food, but those genes are not destined to control your life. That's because there is a difference between the *presence* of genes and their *expression*. Having a set of blueprints in a library does not mean the designs contained within them will ever be used to build something; the same is true of genes. In other words, just having certain genes doesn't mean that those genes will be *expressed*, or 'read' in order to create a functional product.

For a long time, scientists influenced by Darwin's theories believed that inherited genetic changes, or mutations, occur very slowly over hundreds of thousands of years. These mutations are passed from generation to generation and spread very gradually throughout the larger population. Changes that occur during a person's lifetime, however, such as becoming overweight, supposedly could not be passed on to succeeding generations because they do not alter a person's DNA.

New scientific discoveries have dramatically shifted our understanding of genetics. We now know that some changes that occur in a person's lifetime *can*, in fact, be passed on to the next generation or the next several generations. Researchers at Duke University performed a simple experiment in 2006 that showed that the genetic code is more malleable than we realized. They examined a group of mice that carry a specific gene, the agouti gene. An agouti mouse can grow up overweight and sick, or thin and healthy. This depends on the activity of one particular gene during the mouse's gestation. If that gene is silenced and consequently dimmed—the mouse grows up healthy, with a brown coat and a lean body. If the gene is not silenced but remains turned on, the mouse grows a light yellow coat, eats larger quantities of food, and is prone to both diabetes and cancer.

The researchers at Duke changed the diet of yellow-coated mother agouti mice during pregnancy. The added nutrients somehow dimmed the effects of the agouti gene, which enabled the mother to give birth to healthier, leaner babies. These offspring were less likely to grow up to be obese adults. They had normal appetites, even though they still had the agouti gene! It was as if their agouti gene and its effects had been erased from their bodies, yet nothing in their genetic code had changed. On the *genetic* level they were still pure agouti, but on a *functional* level they were not - all because of what their mothers ate. This experiment provided clear evidence that we can change the way genes are expressed, even without altering the genetic code. Such changes can even alter expression in future generations.

Scientists struggled to reconcile this new knowledge with established genetic theory. They realized that while the blueprint for a building is unchanging and must be followed to the tiniest specifications, our DNA blueprint is only partially fixed. Some parts of it are unalterable—for example, the size of our feet—but other parts are more like 'suggestions' or 'possibilities' than true, set-in-stone orders. These parts are highly malleable and quite responsive to the environment, to our emotions, and to what we eat.

Epigenetics

Epigenetics is the study of how people's environments and experiences affect the function and expression of genes. Genes are not just proteins that manufacture a product in a uniform way. They carry chemical attachments that act on the DNA to regulate the timing and amount of the protein without changing its basic composition. These add-ons, or epigenetic markers, evolve as an animal adapts to its environment. A methyl group, composed of a carbon atom bonded with three hydrogen atoms, is an example of an epigenetic marker. When enough methyl groups attach to a gene, they can turn the gene off. On the other hand, if the gene is attached to enough groups of acetyl—another epigenetic marker that includes two carbons, one oxygen and three hydrogen atoms—the gene is switched on. In this way, the genetic code is continually being rewritten.

Who rewrites your epigenetic code? To a large extent you do. You do so every day by eating what you eat, responding to stress the way you do, and otherwise interacting with your environment in your own unique way. The results may affect not only you, but also your unborn children.

Reversing the long-held theory that genes are unalterable prescriptions that dictate not only the color of our eyes but also the diseases we will develop, epigenetics shows that the environment—including our own attitudes, beliefs, life experiences, and behaviors, as well as the time and conditions in which we live—has a great influence over the expression of the genes we were born with.

In this exciting new field, many scientists now study how the environment works to turn genes on and off or make their influence either strong or weak. One of the pioneers of this new field, Dr. Lars Olov Bygren at the Karolinska Institute in Stockholm, studied the effect of years of famine in a remote area of Sweden during the nineteenth century. By early 2000, it was clear to him that the patterns of famine and feast not only powerfully affected the men who had survived them, but also the genetic characteristics of the next generation. Those men who went from famine to feast within a single season, for instance, produced children who lived significantly shorter lives. Bygren's study revealed that these changes in gene activity did not alter the genetic code itself but were still passed down to the next generation.

This growing understanding of epigenetics has profound implications. It overturns the old view that we are prisoners of our genes. The *epigenome*, a term which refers to the full complement of heritable changes to an organism's genome that modify gene expression but *do not* alter the DNA sequence itself, can alter gene expression both negatively and positively. Lifestyle choices like eating too much or not enough, or smoking, for instance, do not only put our own health at risk. These behaviors can also predispose our children to disease and early death.

The National Institutes of Health (NIH) is currently sponsoring over one hundred studies to explore the relationship between epigenetic markers and behavior problems. Some research focuses specifically on obesity. A study of survivors of the Dutch "Hunger Winter", a time of starvation in the Netherlands in the winter of 1944–45, shows that the nutritional status of a woman during pregnancy dramatically influences whether or not her children will ultimately become overweight. When the Germans blockaded the western part of Holland and prevented the Dutch from receiving adequate food, people sometimes had as few as five hundred calories to eat in a day. Fifty years later, infants conceived during the time food was most scarce weighed an average of fourteen pounds or more, had larger waists, and faced a threefold higher risk of coronary artery disease than those whose mothers were further along in their pregnancies when the famine occurred. Researchers found that an important gene for growth during pregnancy was less methylated—or more turned on—in people who were conceived during the worst of the starvation. This study provided the first hard evidence that early life conditions can cause lifelong epigenetic changes in weight.

A recent study of overweight Canadian mothers who gave birth both before and then after weight loss surgery determined that the children born after surgery were half as likely to become overweight as the children born before the surgery.

These studies reveal how environmental influences can lead to epigenetic changes that increase the likelihood of weight gain. But the ability to influence genetic expression also has exciting and empowering implications. A healthy lifestyle can make a difference not only for you, but also for your progeny. Epigenetics shows that even things we can't see—like beliefs, feelings, and attitudes—play an important role in the epigenetic control of our genes, making possible actual changes in cell structure. Scientists are now learning how to manipulate the epigenome to silence bad genes and spur on the good ones.

Researchers are studying links between nutrition and genetics in an effort to discover exactly how the thousands of substances present in food can influence the epigenome, and how that knowledge can be used to make personalized dietary recommendations. Essentially, these researchers are figuring out how to use nutrition to switch specific genes either on or off. This science is in its infancy, but the promise it holds is tremendous.

Every individual's epigenome makes him or her absolutely, fundamentally unique. Even identical twins who begin life with identical genomes accumulate different epigenetic changes as they progress through life, especially if they have different life experiences and consume different diets. Now that we understand every person is truly unique at the molecular level, medical science can work towards providing personalized medical treatments that will help target an individual's unique traits. We will gradually turn the activity of genes up or down, like making adjustments in the balance of a stereo. This will be personalized medicine at its best.

In fact, genetic testing has slowly been incorporated into many psychiatric practices around the country. Genetic research is a useful tool and almost any physician can order a genetic test for a patient. These simple genetic tests, often done by a saliva collection, can inform clinicians of the most appropriate and effective treatment for the patient based on his or her unique genetic profile by analyzing genetic and biological markers. The results reveal how a patient may respond to different psychiatric treatments and can predict weight gain and appetite disturbances that are associated with psychiatric medications. One biological marker with growing interest in many fields of medicine is the *methlentetrahydrofolate reductase* (MTHFR) gene.

The MTHFR gene is responsible for important biochemical reactions, including the conversion of folic acid into *methyltetrahydrofolate*, or MTHF. This nutrient is involved in mood regulation as well as in appetite control, and those with a *polymorphism* (a variant caused by mutation) in this gene will be at a higher risk for mood-related disorders along with appetite disturbances.

Another biological marker that can be analyzed is the *5-hydroxytryptamine 2C* (5-HT2C) *receptor*. It is one of the three receptor subtypes of the 5-HTC receptor family and is often targeted by antipsychotic drugs to treat psychotic disorders such as schizophrenia and depression. However, beyond its role in treating psychosis, the receptor has also been implicated in the control of appetite and subsequent weight maintenance.

We have long known that genetics plays an important role in predisposing individuals to mood disorders. A meta-analysis published in the

American Journal of Psychiatry cited major depression as a familial disorder that results from genetics along with environmental influences. When you are overwhelmed by life stressors, you may not develop depression, but if you had a family history of depression and are overwhelmed by stress, it is likely you are more susceptible to developing depression. Similarly, there may be a genetic component in your biochemical makeup that predisposes you to disordered eating patterns along with other psychiatric illnesses. When you have a strong family history of disordered eating, depression, or other mood disorders, you are at greater risk of developing these disorders than someone who has no family history of any psychiatric illnesses. Comorbid psychiatric illnesses will be discussed in more detail in the following chapter.

Research has made it clear that some epigenetic switches are faithfully copied when sex cells divide, as well as when sperm and egg combine, thus ensuring that the newly created genome will already be influenced by an epigenome. More epigenetic changes may occur in the womb as the fetus is exposed to differing levels and types of nutrients, chemicals (such as PBA), alcohol, stress hormones generated by the mother's body, and other factors.

You can see the inherited epigenome in action in fruit flies. For example, if one generation of fruit flies is exposed to the antibiotic geldanamycin, these flies will develop odd growths on their eyes—and so will the next thirteen generations of their offspring, even though the subsequent generations were not exposed to geldanamycin and have no changes in their DNA. Similarly, feeding roundworms a certain kind of bacteria can make them small and dumpy, and these physical changes can last forty generations or more!

Whether epigenetic changes are good or bad depends on what each specific epigenetic alteration actually accomplishes. In the case of the agouti mice, inheriting the epigenetic "switch" that turns *off* the "overeating and obesity gene" is very helpful. Researchers from Rutgers University discovered that EGCG (epigallocatechin-3-gallate), one of the active ingredients in green tea, prevented epigenetic changes to certain cancer-fighting genes. Preventing these epigenetic changes allowed the cancer-fighting genes to remain active and prevented cancer from growing and spreading. But some epigenetic alterations can also increase the risk of disease. For example, the bacteria *Helicobacter pylori*, which is implicated in ulcers, can trigger epigenetic changes in the digestive tract that may lead to cancer. Abnormal epigenetic markers have been identified in a number of different cancers, including those of the breast, prostate, cervix, and stomach.

We can now see how the epigenome is created and how it influences an individual's life, as well as the lives of offspring, sometimes for multiple generations. Unfortunately, we have not yet been able to identify a single epigenetic change that leads to disordered eating, and we cannot zero in on a medicine, diet or other approach that will reverse that change.

What we *can* do is to set the stage for a helpful rather than a harmful epigenome by examining genetic markers like MTHFR, consuming a nutritious diet, reducing stress, and otherwise giving the body the tools it needs to build good health. At the same time, we can avoid dangerous habits and behaviors that might set up a deleterious change in the epigenome—a change that may be passed on to the next generation and beyond.

Our genes provide the blueprints for who we may become; they do not, however, determine who we are. As we learn more about how each person is both unique and extraordinary, we will also be able to provide effective help because such help will be specifically, biochemically tailored to the individual. We must treat patients for coexisting conditions that exacerbate appetite problems. Understanding an individual's genetic vulnerabilities and genetic makeup will allow us to personalize treatment recommendations. This is part of the New Hope, and it leads the way off the roller coaster.

Summary

All individuals are unique and extraordinary in their own right. Not only does obvious individuality exist when it comes to appearance and personality, but within each of us are profound biochemical differences that shape our experiences. Genes are the blueprints of the body and mind that create these varying traits—the instructions that determine the distinct form and function of all the cells in the body. Passed down through generations and combined uniquely at birth, genes create a diversity of physical, behavioral, and biochemical characteristics.

Many studies have demonstrated a clear link between genetics and a predisposition to weight gain and addictive behaviors. However, while it was once believed that genes programmed the body unalterably, newer research has shown that different factors—including the times and locations we live in as well as our attitudes and beliefs—can greatly influence the expression of genes. This is *epigenetics*, the study of cellular and physiologic trait variations caused by external or environmental factors that can switch genes 'on' or 'off' or alter their expression. New information derived from cutting-edge epigenetic research is greatly helpful to clinicians, who can use genetic information and biomarkers to formulate effective, personalized treatment plans that target specific vulnerabilities. Moreover, epigenetics empowers us to know that the choices we make daily can have an impact on our sustained health and happiness, and to recognize that there is a way off the roller coaster of disordered eating.

Key Points

- Everyone is unique not only in personality and appearance, but also in intricate biochemical differences in anatomy and metabolism.
- Genes are the blueprints of the body and mind. They are passed on through generations and combined in a unique way at birth to determine the form and function of all the cells in the body.
- Research has defined a clear relationship between genetics and a predisposition to food addiction, taste, and weight gain.
- Epigenetics is the study of how environmental factors, attitudes, beliefs, and experiences affect the expression of the genes we are born with.

- Researchers are studying the link between nutrition and genetics and how certain substances in food can influence the epigenome.
- Genetic mutations such as MTHFR polymorphisms can cause appetite disturbances, and testing is now available to analyze these biomedical markers.
- Epigenetic research and genetic testing are useful tools that will help clinicians decide on the most effective treatment by analyzing a patient's unique genetic and biological markers.

5
COMPREHENSIVE EVALUATIONS FOR APPETITE CONTROL

One of the most common problems I see in the treatment of disordered eating is the failure to diagnose and treat coexisting psychiatric disorders that affect mood, emotions, and behaviors. Before looking at food and appetite as problems in and of themselves, it's important to explore the entire context of disordered eating—that is, to discover whether there is a co-occurring disorder intertwined with and reinforcing unhealthy eating patterns.

Whenever I evaluate a new patient with an eating disorder, I try to learn about the interplay between his or her disordered eating and other psychiatric conditions. For instance, a patient with an untreated mood disorder such as depression may be using food to self-medicate. Or a patient with a family history of alcoholism may have a biochemical tendency to engage in the kind of impulsive behavior manifest in bingeing and purging. If these psychiatric conditions or genetic predispositions exist, they will hijack a patient's efforts to control appetite and weight management until they are successfully treated.

The coexistence of biologically-based psychiatric diagnoses and appetite problems is common. One research study concluded that approximately eighty percent of patients with binge eating disorder (BED) and ninety-five percent of patients with bulimia met the criteria for at least one other diagnosis outlined in the *Diagnostic and Statistical Manual of Mental Disorders*. Overweight men and women are twenty-five percent more likely to suffer from mood disorders than the rest of the population. Some research suggests that up to three-quarters of people with eating disorders also have depression. Ten percent of people with eating disorders have coexisting bipolar disorder and forty percent show signs of obsessive-compulsive disorder (OCD). Between fifteen percent and forty percent of patients with eating disorders also struggle with substance abuse.

Coexisting Attention-Deficit Hyperactivity Disorder (ADHD)

Attention-deficit/hyperactivity disorder (ADHD) is a medical condition associated with difficulty concentrating, staying organized, and controlling impulses. Although people with this diagnosis may appear to be bursting with energy, they have trouble channeling that energy effectively and controlling their impulsivity. They may act before they have thought things through, speak out of turn, or say things they later regret. Because of poor planning, missed appointments, and forgotten details, both personal and work relationships may suffer.

Our culture bombards us with enticements for high-calorie food, which makes it difficult for individuals who eat in reaction to environmental cues (as opposed to the sensation of hunger) to eat healthily and in accordance with natural hunger signals. People suffering from ADHD and people with disordered eating deal with boredom, stress, and intense feelings by overeating in order to soothe themselves. Those with ADHD may be particularly likely to forget to eat and to binge later. Or they may have trouble planning and shopping ahead, which can result in spur-of-the-moment and uncontrolled eating.

Considerable recent research focuses on connections between ADHD and overeating in adolescents and adults. One study reported a twelve percent prevalence rate of ADHD amongst women with bulimia compared to a prevalence rate of zero to two percent in a control group of healthy women. In a 2009 study published in the *Journal of Psychiatric Research*, the authors found that symptoms of ADHD are significantly elevated in overweight adults both with and without binge eating, suggesting that ADHD screening should be conducted on patients seeking treatment for obesity and binge eating.

A recent study conducted by researchers at the Child Study Center at New York University's Langone Medical Center found that men who were diagnosed with ADHD as children were twice as likely to be overweight in a thirty-three-year follow-up study compared to those who were not diagnosed with the condition. Results from the study show that men with childhood ADHD had a significantly higher body mass index, or BMI (30.1 versus 27.6) and obesity rates (41.1% versus 21.6%). The researchers attributed the higher incidence of obesity occurring in adults with ADHD to lack of impulse control and poor planning skills, leading to poor food choices and irregular eating habits. Children and adolescents with ADHD need to be taught healthy eating habits in order to avoid developing disordered eating patterns.

In a study published in November of 2013, researchers explored the psychiatric manifestations of ADHD in patients with binge eating and found a positive association between the frequency of binge episodes and the level of ADHD symptoms among 191 female participants. The results were consistent with many other studies citing a correlation between disordered eating and ADHD. Individuals with ADHD tend to have personalities characterized by high novelty seeking and low self-directedness, which increases the severity of the disordered eating behavior.

Another research study of 215 patients in treatment for weight problems found a strikingly high prevalence of ADHD: 27.4%. Among those with obesity, the prevalence of ADHD was a staggering 42.6%. Because women with ADHD are often not hyperactive, their ADHD is often unrecognized. Consequently, they don't receive the early treatment for ADHD that could also help them overcome disordered eating.

Like depression and anxiety, ADHD is now viewed by experts as being caused by an imbalance in brain chemistry. The neurotransmitters *norepinephrine* and dopamine may be in short supply in the brains of those with ADHD. Although too much norepinephrine can contribute to anxiety, too little can cause problems with concentration and learning. Those with a deficiency in norepinephrine have trouble blocking out distractions and organizing their lives.

Dopamine is essential for the control of impulses and for enabling a person to sit still and wait. Animals in the wild freeze in their tracks in response to a threat because of a blast of dopamine. People who lack act impulsively, blurt out opinions, and burst out in anger (often feeling regret later). As dopamine is an essential part of the body's reward circuit, a deficiency in this neurotransmitter intensifies the urge to indulge in behaviors such as overeating, substance abuse, and other risk-taking behaviors to achieve the same reward sensations that others may experience from less harmful behaviors. People whose brains are low in dopamine often self-medicate with high-caloric food because of its ability to activate dopamine in the common reward pathway.

A deficiency in the two neurotransmitters norepinephrine and dopamine can lead to the following eating-related behaviors:

- Poor awareness of internal cues of hunger and satiety (fullness)
- Inability to follow a meal plan
- Inability to judge portion size accurately
- Inability to stop bingeing or purging
- Distraction by continual thoughts of food, weight and body shape
- Increased desire to overeat, especially high-calorie, "reward" type foods
- Poor self-esteem due to repeated failures at self-control

In patients with coexisting psychiatric and eating problems, which came first? Is ADHD the switch that turns on disordered eating, or does the eating disorder leave the brain so undernourished that it can't function optimally? Just what precedes what appears to vary depending on the individual: in some, eating disturbances evolve concurrently with other psychiatric symptoms; in others, signs of a psychiatric disorder are not apparent until the disordered eating patterns are firmly established. In still others, problems with mood and problems with appetite seem to have always coexisted. Regardless of the order of onset, the simultaneous presence of disordered eating and a mental illness means that effective treatment for the disordered eating must address *both* conditions. This is the only approach that will slowly lead the way to recovery and prevent the all-too-common patterns of relapse and repeated failures.

The relationship between many psychiatric disorders with disordered eating is complex. ADHD is the most commonly missed diagnosis in relation to food and appetite problems. All adults seeking treatment for binge eating or obesity should be screened for ADHD. I believe effective treatment for ADHD can significantly help patients off the roller coaster of disordered eating.

Fortunately, I have witnessed many times a dramatic reduction in disordered eating once a patient is treated for ADHD. The strong urge to binge or to self-medicate with food subsides once the impulsivity and inattention of ADHD are treated. The individual experiences a new ability to tune in to his or her body's signals, control cravings, and improve impulse control.

Coexisting Depression

Everyone experiences sadness; it is an inevitable accompaniment to losses in life and part of the range of emotions that make us human. Depression, however, is different, as it involves many more symptoms than just a sad mood. Depression is defined as a consistently low mood for a period of two weeks or more. Patients with major depression usually have a markedly different mood from their usual state of mind, and their functioning is impaired. They may lose joy in their hobbies and interests, experience difficulty sleeping and concentrating, and think frequently about death and suicide.

Strikingly, seventy-five percent of patients with eating disorders also suffer from depression. For those individuals with binge eating disorder who are also overweight, one study found that rates of depression are even higher than for individuals who are overweight but do not have binge eating disorder. In this particular study, researchers found that symptoms of depression led to binge eating episodes. Other studies have found that depressive symptoms, including low self-esteem, predicted increases in binge eating, demonstrating further evidence of the relationship between depression and binge eating. These results suggest that binge eating for some is a way to regulate emotion. It seems clear that the treatment of any underlying mood disorders is critical to the treatment of binge eating disorder.

Depression and binge eating disorder result from alterations in neurotransmitters, which relay messages from one brain cell to another and then to the rest of the body. We know that imbalances in any of the neurotransmitters can wreak havoc with brain circuitry. Normal levels of *serotonin*, a neurotransmitter linked to feelings of well-being, happiness, and satisfaction, lead both to emotional satisfaction and a sense of fullness after a meal. Low levels, on the other hand, can lead to depression and a tendency to binge on sweet and starchy foods. In fact, one study looking at how depression and a gene associated with lower levels of serotonin related to binge eating found that depressed children and older females who carried this gene were more likely to engage in binge eating behaviors. Low serotonin is one of the links between depression and disordered eating. In Chapters 9 and 11, we will discuss how amino acids and medications can support and enhance serotonin synthesis.

Coexisting Anxiety

Anxiety is unfounded worry or exaggerated fears. While fear is a healthy response to real or impending danger, anxiety is an excessive response to a danger that might not even exist. For example, anxiety can motivate someone afraid of causing a motor vehicle crash to avoid driving.

Anxiety can develop into an *anxiety disorder*, an umbrella term for a number of different disorders which include panic disorder, generalized anxiety disorder, phobias, post-traumatic stress disorder (PTSD), and OCD.

Obsessive-compulsive disorder is commonly found in eating disorder patients, as those suffering from an eating disorder frequently obsess about food, body image, and food preparation, and feel uncontrollably compelled to engage in unhealthy eating behaviors. An increasing number of women are actually obsessed about healthy, "clean" eating, which is called *orthorexia nervosa*—essentially a preoccupation with avoiding foods considered to be unhealthy.

The current and lifetime prevalence rates of OCD are higher in people with eating disorders than in the general population. The greater number of OCD traits you exhibit as a child, the more likely you are to develop an eating disorder. A diagnosis of OCD often precedes the diagnosis of an eating disorder, indicating that eating disorders may develop as a way of coping with anxiety.

Bingeing may be a coping mechanism for many individuals who suffer from PTSD. There is a strong link between childhood abuse and trauma and eating disorders. Studies have revealed a strong correlation between a history of childhood emotional abuse and *bulimia spectrum disorders* (BSD). A 2012 Montreal study of 176 women with BSD and 139 without current or past eating disorders found that bulimia spectrum disorders correlated with childhood emotional abuse at a significantly higher rate than with physical or sexual abuse, at 80.7% versus 41.6% and 25%, respectively. This study corroborates a 2010 survey of 489 university women that found early childhood abuse was the most consistent predictor of bulimia.

Early childhood abuse can help us predict eating pathology and can influence an individual's eating behavior later in life. Many of you who have suffered early childhood abuse may be using food as a compensatory mechanism to help cope with the trauma. Addressing underlying issues will allow you to break free from disordered eating. I will discuss in Chapter 15 the value of therapy to augment medications or nutritional support and to help you regain control of your appetite and eating patterns.

Anxiety can manifest itself in various kinds of disturbances with eating. A compulsive dieter tries to exert control over her life and soothe her nerves by severely restricting her food intake. Then there is the person who binges then diets, fights the urge to eat, and keeps track of every bite until she gives in to her escalating anxiety and eats without restraint. The person whose disordered eating follows a pattern of bingeing and purging becomes so anxious about what she's eaten during a binge that she purges – not merely as a way to relieve herself of calories but also as a way to relieve guilt and anxiety. Recurring thoughts about food, eating, weight, and self-worth can trigger underlying anxiety that contributes to disordered eating patterns.

Scientific research has repeatedly demonstrated a high correlation between anxiety disorders and eating disorders. Anxiety disorders most commonly associated with eating disorders include obsessive-compulsive disorder, social phobia, generalized anxiety disorder, and panic disorder. Many of you may use binge eating as a compensatory mechanism to help decrease anxiety. The flood of endorphins from binge eating floods your brain with chemical changes that temporarily provide neurochemical relief from emotional distress and anxiety. Ultimately, however, this coping mechanism usually fails.

Since two-thirds of people with an eating disorder have had an anxiety disorder diagnosed prior to the development of their eating disorder, it is critical to treat the underlying anxiety disorders that may exacerbate disordered eating.

Coexisting Substance Abuse

Perhaps the most challenging problem that tends to coexist with disordered eating is substance abuse. Between fifteen percent and forty percent of patients with eating disorders also struggle with substance abuse. The connection between food and addiction is such a critical aspect of disordered eating that I have devoted a chapter in this book to exploring the subject more fully. I mention it here because substance abuse is the most complex to treat of the problems that can be intertwined with disordered eating.

Dependence on an addictive substance such as alcohol or a narcotic drug works through the body's reward circuit. This brain pathway is powered by dopamine, which increases desire, and serotonin, which increases satiety and inhibition. This brain pathway creates an incentive to engage in certain advantageous behaviors, such as eating, quenching your thirst, or having sex. And whether the objective is indeed obtaining food, a drink of water, or sexual relations, the pathway works in essentially the same way. When you engage in these behaviors, your body responds by generating good feelings that make you want to repeat the behaviors. However, the circuit also generates rewards in response to non-desirable behaviors, such as the abuse of food, alcohol, heroin, cocaine, amphetamines, and nicotine.

While cocaine and amphetamines act directly on the brain cells that produce dopamine and alcohol and heroin affect them indirectly, all of these substances increase dopamine release as a reward, at least initially. However, many dopamine receptors may "die off" due to over-use, leading to a lessening of dopamine activity. The brain can't get dopamine in high enough amounts because there aren't enough receptors. This means that larger amounts of the substance of abuse will be needed to produce the same feeling. A pattern of substance abuse wreaks havoc with the brain's reward circuits and dims the mental faculties responsible for making judgments and postponing gratification. It is nearly impossible to break a pattern of disordered eating without first or simultaneously treating substance abuse issues.

Summary

Disordered eating patterns often occur in tandem with other biologically-based psychiatric disorders that have an impact on mood, emotions, and behaviors. In order to recover from food addiction and restore appetite, you must receive concurrent treatment for all existing mental conditions. Depression is the most common coexisting diagnosis in individuals struggling with appetite regulation, as both diagnoses result from imbalances in neurotransmitters. Anxiety and related disorders such as OCD and PTSD, which typically involve social phobias, distorted body image, and compulsions related to food, are also closely correlated. Attention-deficit hyperactivity disorder has a strong and often overlooked connection with eating disorders, stemming from shared characteristics such as increased susceptibility to environmental stimuli, low self-esteem, chaotic eating patterns, and dopamine imbalance. Substance abuse can also be intertwined with disordered eating due to similar biochemical shifts and addictive patterns. If you suspect that an underlying anxiety or mood disorder is causing or exacerbating disordered eating, it is important to work with a qualified physician or mental health practitioner who can help guide you to the most comprehensive and successful care.

Key Points

- It is common for those with disordered eating to have coexisting biological psychiatric disorders that affect mood, emotions, and behaviors.
- Depression is the diagnosis most frequently associated with disordered eating. Both result from changes in the function of neurotransmitters; specifically, low serotonin.
- Anxiety and related disorders, including OCD and PTSD, are correlated with eating disorders. Overlapping traits include feeling compelled to eat, preoccupations with food preparation, social phobias, panic, and altered body image.
- ADHD is strongly associated with disrupted eating patterns and obesity, yet it is often undiagnosed. Shared characteristics include chaotic eating habits, distorted body image, low self-esteem, dopamine imbalance, and increased susceptibility to environmental stimuli.
- Substance abuse and food addiction result from a similar disruption in the reward centers of the brain.
- For a successful recovery from eating and appetite problems, there must be simultaneous treatment of other existing mental conditions.

6
FOOD ADDICTION: THE SCIENCE OF SUGAR

For most of us, happy associations with sugar are part of the culture we inherited. "Sugar" is a term of endearment. Little girls are made of "sugar and spice/and everything nice." Sugar helps us cope with the painful realities of life. To make it more palatable, we may "sugar-coat" a difficult truth. As Mary Poppins, Julie Andrews cheerfully sang, "A spoonful of sugar helps the medicine go down." Joseph Sabin surely became the patron saint of childhood when he devised a way to replace the dreaded polio injection with an oral dose that children could take in a sugar cube. You may remember cookies in a jar in your mother's kitchen. And, of course, beyond these positive emotional memories, sugar tastes great. A sugary treat is often a reward; it gives a quick boost of energy and, usually, a smile.

It's hard to face the fact that despite these pleasant images and our individual attachments to favorite desserts, sugar, for some, is an addictive drug. It functions in the body in ways similar to those of other addictive drugs—alcohol, morphine and cocaine. Its power to hijack our bodies' reward systems leads Gayle King, host of *CBS This Morning*, to confess, "Krispy Kreme is like heroin to me."

Sugar Is Everywhere

Paradoxically, the damage that sugar inflicts in our society is often difficult to see. . .because sugar is everywhere. Our children commonly and regularly consume excessive amounts of sugar. For many, the effects of sugar overconsumption accumulate so gradually that we have become inured to their devastating consequences.

Sugar used to be a rare treat in America. Its use has increased a staggering 330% since colonial days. In 1700, American colonists averaged four pounds of sugar a year. By the year 1800, Americans were eating eighteen pounds per year. At the turn of another century, in 1900, the average American consumed ninety pounds of sugar annually. The advent of food processing boosted the food industry's capacity to package sugary treats that could stay on the supermarket shelves for months without diminishing their appeal. The Hostess Twinkie, introduced in 1930, was among the first of these fast food treats, and it was anything but rare. By 1980, Americans' per capita sugar consumption had reached one hundred and twenty pounds. By 2010, that amount had escalated to 132 pounds per year.

We have now become accustomed to turning to sugar for a quick mood lift and boost of energy. The taste for sugar can even develop in utero. Doctors used to treat the problem of excessive amniotic fluid by injecting a sweet substance in the uterus. This prompted the fetus to swallow more fluid, which was flushed through the umbilical cord and out through the mother's kidneys. Infants prefer sweet tastes. Drinking a sugar solution eases pain through a natural analgesic effect. A positive early-life association with sugar sets the stage for a lifelong relationship, not only with sweet-tasting foods that we all associate with sugar, like chocolate chip cookies and cheesecake, but in a surprising range of savory foods and even nonfood items: browned vegetables, yogurt, ketchup, canned soup, bread, bacon, bologna, crackers, soy sauce, French fries, margarine, pretzels, lip gloss and toothpaste.

The Dangers of Sugar

Foods rich in sugar at first cause blood glucose levels to soar—leading to a surge of insulin. *Insulin* is the hormone that ferries glucose into cells to produce energy or to be stored in fat cells. When insulin clears too much glucose, blood sugar drops, precipitating both a decline in mood and a craving for more sugar. Then you crave sugar again, leading to more insulin release and soaring blood glucose. This cycle can eventually lead to a phenomenon known as *insulin resistance*. The insulin "key" no longer "unlocks" the cells, less glucose can be taken in, and the cells starve. When cells resist the effects of insulin, blood levels of both insulin and glucose rise. The highs and lows of the cycle become magnified: an abnormally high glucose spike is followed by an abnormally low glucose drop. Repetition and escalation of this cycle eventually cause an increase in blood fats, triglycerides, and cholesterol. Sugar cravings can become irresistible. The blood sugar crash in turn affects the adrenal glands, which push the blood sugar level back up by releasing adrenaline, which then stimulates another hormone called *cortisol*. This hormone triggers intense cravings for sugar. The spiral continues.

Many scientists believe that the increase in the amount of sugar we consume as a species has fueled the multitude of obesity and diabetes epidemics that are ongoing worldwide. In 1890, white American males in their fifties had an obesity rate of 3.4%. By 1980, the rate had reached fifteen percent; it has more than doubled since then. Seventy percent of Americans are now overweight. In 1980, 5.5% of American children were overweight; by 2010, that percentage had reached an alarming 16.9%. The Organization for Economic Cooperation and Development (OECD) recently established that the United States is the fattest nation of thirty-three countries they studied. The increase in the rate of diabetes in the United States parallels our nation's increase in sugar consumption. It has nearly tripled in a generation, from 2.5% in 1980 to 6.8% in 2010.

Sugar Is Addictive

Sugar acts on the brain to disrupt normal neurochemical physiology. It interferes with the suppression of the hormone *ghrelin*, which signals hunger to the brain and which is normally dampened after a big meal.

Sugar blocks the transport of the hormone *leptin*, which contributes to the feeling of fullness. Sugar also weakens dopamine signaling in the brain's reward center, which lies at the root of its capacity to fuel addiction-like symptoms that disrupt normal controls for appetite regulation.

Researchers have learned about the biological bases of food addiction by studying animal behavior and neurochemistry. The study of rats has yielded an astonishing wealth of insight, particularly research into the effects of sugar consumption on dopamine levels in rats' brains. When researchers provide rats with access to a sugar solution, the rats' brains release dopamine. This fuels a need to consume more. Over time, the rats' brains adapt to increased dopamine levels, triggering increasingly-urgent cravings for yet more sugar. The desire for sweetness is so urgent that the rats even prefer sugar water to cocaine. Even rats *already addicted to cocaine* consistently choose sugar above all else.

When the sugar water is then withdrawn from the cages, the rats show signs of anxiety and physical dependence. Normally, rats tend to explore their environments. Rats withdrawing from sugar, however, refuse to venture into an open part of their maze and instead remain huddled in a tunnel. Withdrawal makes them too anxious to explore; their teeth chatter, and they startle easily.

Giving rats a sugar solution on an intermittent basis as opposed to regularly accelerates their urge to consume it. Indeed, lab rats with limited access to sugar essentially eat themselves to death. They will walk across an electrified plate and choose to undergo shocks in order to get their fix. One study showed that rats with limited access to sucrose—one hour per day—would gradually consume sixty-five percent of their calories for the day in one sitting. Even if they later were fed regular chow after the sugar was withdrawn, these rats withdrew into the fetal position, twitching. Their body temperatures lowered. The tremors and shakes these rats displayed mirror the effects of withdrawal from narcotics in humans. The researchers concluded that the quantity of sugar consumed and the intermittency of their access to it did, in combination, intensify the power of the rats' physiological sugar addiction.

Researchers have long known that rats with intermittent access to sugar show two of the three elements of addiction: they increase their consumption of sugar water over time, and they show signs of withdrawal when the sucrose is taken away. If the relationship that develops between the rats and sugar is really addictive, scientists have reasoned, there should be observable, long-lasting changes in the rats' brains that ultimately lead to craving and relapse.

The presence of this third element of addiction was verified when lab rats were denied sugar for a period of time after they had gradually learned to binge. The rats worked harder than ever to reach the sucrose when it was reintroduced, and they consumed more than ever before. This would not have occurred unless the neurochemical pathways within the rats' brains had indeed been altered by addiction.

In addition, the changes in their brain chemistry made the rats more susceptible to other forms of addiction. After their sucrose supply was taken from the cage, they consumed more alcohol than they had when exposed previously. This behavior proved to the researchers that the rats' sugar bingeing had actually changed the functioning of their brains. These neurochemical changes served as gateways to other destructive behaviors, including an increased vulnerability to alcohol abuse.

In one study, rats in withdrawal from sugar consumption were given a low dose of amphetamine. The dose was in fact so low that normally it would produce no measurable effect, but these rats became hyperactive. The outcome of this study confirmed the researchers' conclusion that sugar had changed the rats' brain function. A heightened sensitivity to stimulant drugs was a lasting brain alteration that resulted from sugar addiction. The brain was changed by the food addiction cycle of withdrawal and reward. Behavioral changes arising from sugar addiction parallel the brain changes documented in morphine- or alcohol-dependent rats.

The neurochemical changes in sugar-addicted rats are identical to those observed in humans. After high sugar intake, the human brain is flooded with dopamine. It compensates for the overabundance by decreasing the total number of dopamine receptors, which means the brain cannot continue to utilize dopamine efficiently. This "down regulation" means that the activity of receptors in the limbic system, the site of motivation and emotions, is dampened.

After this down regulation, the brain demands greater and greater amounts of sugary foods in order to achieve the same dopamine rush. Ironically, the more you feed the craving, the less satisfaction you feel. Each time the brain is flooded, additional dopamine receptors are affected. As these receptors disappear, the effect of dopamine upon the prefrontal cortex is also diminished. This is the part of the brain that gets you to put aside short-term pleasure in favor of long-term gain. Just as your cells are getting hungrier for more dopamine, the signal from the prefrontal cortex is easily drowned out by the desire for more. This is the biology behind a fundamental truth that has long perplexed the doctors and family members of alcoholics and other drug addicts: you *cannot* reason an addict out of his addiction. The part of the addict's brain that reasons and understands consequences is held hostage by another part - the primitive and powerful reward center of the brain.

Nora Volkow, Director of the National Institute of Drug Abuse (NIDA), has participated in extensive research assessing the connection between sugar and addiction. To study how foods hijack the brain's reward system, she has used radioactive chemicals that bind to dopamine receptors in combination with *positron emission tomography* (PET) scans. Her research has shown that overweight people have far fewer dopamine receptors in their brain's reward centers and, therefore, have to eat more food in order to achieve the same 'dopamine reward' as individuals of average weight.

Brain imaging technologies provide scientists with tangible confirmation as to sugar's addictive effects. PET scans reveal reactions in the brain to images of palatable foods. A person addicted to sweet foods looks at a picture of a delicious dessert and the corresponding region of the brain lights up in the scan. This is exactly the light pattern visible in the scans of alcoholics. Using *functional magnetic resonance imaging* (fMRI), researchers from Yale showed that both lean and overweight women who test positive for sugar addiction evidence the exact pattern of neural activity that a chronic drug addict displays: high levels of anticipation of the drug of choice—chocolate, in this particular experiment—and low satisfaction after eating.

These researchers have found many similarities between the effects of sugar and drugs commonly recognized as addictive. The same reward-related neuronal activity can be observed in both food addiction and other substance dependence. Food restriction, a common behavior of binge eaters and bulimics early in the day, enhances the reinforcing effect of both sugar and drugs like cocaine and alcohol.

Without being aware of it, the minds of many individuals who struggle with disordered eating are controlled by neurochemical processes that take place when they eat sugar. Whereas rats will walk across electrified plates and subject themselves to shocks in order to get sugar, we may persist in subjecting ourselves to catastrophic consequences—obesity, low self-esteem, deteriorating health, or chronic, out-of-control behaviors—just to get our next fix. Like addictive drugs, sugar triggers neurobiological adaptations that make behavior increasingly compulsive. We fight what seems a losing battle to gain control. Like the rat in the cage, we may be stuck on the treadmill, unable to get off.

The Truth Will Come Out

If sugar is so dangerous, why have so many western cultures been so slow to acknowledge this fact? In the early twentieth century, dentist Weston A. Price traveled the world from the territories of the Inuit in his native Canada to the far South Seas. In 1939 he published *Nutrition and Physical Degeneration: A Comparison of Primitive and Modern Diets and Their Effects*, in which he observed that people who live in ways and under conditions that most westerners would label 'primitive' had excellent teeth and superior general health. They ate natural, unrefined foods sourced from their homelands. As soon as refined, sugary foods were introduced via contacts with western civilizations, Dr. Price concluded, physical degeneration in these native peoples became obvious within a single generation.

Dr. Price's work did not receive the immediate attention it deserved. Although *The New York Times* labeled sugar "a villain in disguise" and compared its effects to those of cigarettes and alcohol in 1977, the sugar industry quickly mobilized arguments discounting this conclusion. Research into the links that the article proposed do exist between sugar and chronic disease was virtually nonexistent. The industry argued that sugar is healthy - because it is present in nature.

In fact, the sugar industry's successful efforts to block public awareness of the dangers of sugar constitute a story of intrigue and manipulation. The nation's meteoric increase in sugar consumption coincided with the industry's efforts to maintain the image of sugar as innocuous and unfairly demeaned by "health food kooks." The sugar industry kept alive a sense of uncertainty about sugar's true health effects, and protected its sales by creating a body of evidence that companies could use to counter any damaging research. In the 1970s and 1980s, the Sugar Association designed studies to support the industry's defense. Each proposal was reviewed by a scientific panel friendly to the industry as well as a committee staffed by representatives of companies like Coca-Cola, Hershey, General Mills, and Nabisco. The industry has fought through the decades to prevent the US Department of Agriculture and the Food and Drug Administration from setting recommended limits on sugar consumption.

In 2012, Robert Lustig, an endocrinologist and a specialist in pediatric obesity at the University of California–San Francisco, called the recent worldwide spike in sugar consumption "the biggest public health crisis in the history of the world." He predicts that the truth scientists have now demonstrated as to sugar's power to trigger biological addiction will follow the same path as the scientific truth about the dangers of nicotine. We know how the nicotine story ended: at long last, those who made money from Big Tobacco had to concede that cigarettes are dangerous and addictive. Lustig observes, "The science is in and the sugar industry may be facing the inexorable exposure of sugar as a killer." But, he concludes, "Even the inexorable can be held up for a very long time."

There is no need for us to wait. The science shows clearly that sugar is one of the most significant villains fueling the food addiction epidemic that has become so prevalent in our society. Drastically reducing sugar in the diet will break the cycle of craving, reward, and withdrawal that keeps us out of control.

Intense sugar cravings are usually brought on by high-carbohydrate diets. Many individuals find relief from sugar cravings when their diets are adjusted to be low in carbohydrates and processed foods. If you reintroduce too many carbohydrates into your diet, you will experience an increase in sugar cravings and an urge to eat, even if you are not hungry. While I am not advocating that you eliminate carbohydrates from your diet *completely*, it may be worthwhile to *reduce* your overall carbohydrate intake. You will be surprised to find that you experience cravings less often. Eventually, as nutritional support and therapy are integrated into treatment, you will find more freedom in adjusting the balance of carbohydrates in your diet. A licensed dietician can help you understand the importance of a balanced diet.

Summary

Sugar is ubiquitous in many western cultures. It is sprinkled onto plates as aesthetic decoration, it is celebrated in song, it is immortalized in turns of phrase, sayings, and stories, and it is worked into the very fabric of our memories. With the wild increase in consumption of processed convenience foods and beverages that has occurred in westernized countries over the past century, we as a species are now eating more sugar than we have in the entirety of our history. Although spoken of innocently, sugar is one of the most significant and dangerous contributors to disordered eating due to its highly addictive nature and its disruptive health effects.

The body is simply not adapted to deal with an overabundance of sugar. When an excess of sugar is ingested, blood levels of glucose rise and dip dramatically. This fluctuation creates a destabilizing hormone cycle that creates addictive cravings and disrupts natural appetite cues. The functions of leptin and ghrelin—the hormones that indicate a sense of hunger and fullness—are blocked in the presence of too much sugar. Eventually, the body's cells become resistant to insulin, the hormone that guides glucose into the cells where it can be used as fuel. Thus, in the phenomenon known as insulin resistance, the body suffers from a surplus of sugar in the blood, while the cells are left malnourished and starving.

Many researchers have suggested that dietary sugar is a major contributor to global obesity epidemics and high incidence rates of diabetes. Reducing sugar consumption is a key step in gaining freedom from cravings, breaking the cycle of food addiction, and stabilizing appetite.

Key Points

- In western cultures, sugar is used for celebration, valued for taste, and cherished as part of tradition.
- Over the past century, global sugar consumption has increased drastically concurrent with the rising popularity of processed foods and beverages.
- Sugar is a major contributor to disordered eating because of its strong emotional associations, addictive qualities, and other negative health consequences.
- Excess sugar destabilizes blood glucose levels, causing damaging spikes and plunges. An erratic pattern of blood glucose disrupts hormone function and creates uncontrollable chemical cravings for more sweet foods.
- When exposed to a continuous sugar surplus, cells eventually develop an insensitivity to insulin, the hormone that guides glucose into cells. When insulin resistance occurs, glucose can no longer reach the cells that need it as a fuel. As a result, the body stays hungry for more and more sugar while cells starve.
- Sugar intake contributes to a rise in blood fats, triglycerides, and cholesterol. Excess glucose is sent to the liver, where it is converted into a fatty acid form and deposited in areas of the body where it can create problems.

- Many researchers suggest that high sugar consumption has fueled the obesity epidemics and high diabetes rates that are increasingly prevalent in westernized cultures.
- Sugar disrupts the appetite mechanism by inhibiting the suppression of the hunger hormone ghrelin and by blocking transport of the hormone leptin, which signals fullness. It also commandeers the brain's reward center by weakening response to the pleasure-creating neurotransmitter dopamine.
- Reducing sugar intake breaks the addictive cycle of craving, reward, and withdrawal, allowing the appetite to stabilize and health to return.

7
FOOD ADDICTION: THE CHEMISTRY OF DAIRY AND WHEAT

I have discussed how sugar can cause symptoms of addiction and affect the ability to control food intake. Binges may begin with sugar, but then may be followed with large quantities of food often containing dairy and wheat. In fact, studies show that when people binge, they gravitate toward carbohydrates such as cakes and crackers, and dairy products like ice cream. There are good reasons we reach for these foods over others during a binge, as both wheat and dairy are broken down into small protein fragments that have effects similar to opiate drugs such as morphine.

The "no gluten" craze has overtaken bookshelves, media outlets, radio stations, and coffee shop discussions. *Wheatophobia* is now heard everywhere; the term describes individuals who avoid wheat in all foods. One frequently-discussed book, *Wheat Belly* by William Davis, explains the addictive potential of wheat and its contribution to current obesity epidemics. Davis assures his readers that eliminating wheat from their diets will lead to weight loss and improved health.

David Perlmutter's new book, *Grain Brain*, discusses his belief that carbohydrates are the cause of almost every modern neurologic disease including dementia, decreased libido, depression, anxiety, headaches, epilepsy, and ADHD. Wheat is not necessarily harmful for everyone, and doesn't always cause bingeing, weight gain, or food cravings; individuals with sensitivities to gluten, however, should avoid wheat, as it can contribute to disordered eating behaviors. We are now able to test for a wide range of physiological abnormalities related to gluten intolerance. Although many patients have abnormal reactions, eliminating gluten is not the answer for everyone struggling with disordered eating. Laboratory testing will confirm any sensitivity to gluten, and the results will motivate you to adopt a stricter diet if a gluten sensitivity is indeed revealed.

Celiac Disease

One type of gluten sensitivity is *celiac disease*, an autoimmune disorder that may be associated with binge eating disorder. Celiac disease is a sensitivity to the *gluten* found in wheat and other grains, meaning that the body mistakenly identifies gluten as a foreign invader and launches an immune attack. Over time, the damage caused by the autoimmune reaction to gluten makes it difficult or impossible for the body to absorb certain nutrients from foods. Digestive problems and nutritional deficiencies are common consequences of untreated celiac disease. In one study, the mortality risk of people with undiagnosed celiac disease over a forty-five-year period was four times higher than that of people without the disease.

In undiagnosed celiac disease, malnutrition and malabsorption can fuel an increased appetite and trigger binge eating episodes along with disordered eating. When your body isn't obtaining an adequate supply of nutrients, it will send signals to your brain to prompt you to eat. Treating underlying nutritional deficiencies will help you avoid disordered eating behaviors. The treatment of celiac disease, however, requires you to avoid all gluten products.

Another peptide implicated in binge eating and disordered eating is *casein*, which is found in dairy products. During normal digestion, both gluten and casein are broken down into amino acids that can then be used to create hormones and neurotransmitters that are essential for a healthy, functioning body. In some people, however, gluten and casein are not broken down into amino acids. The by-products of this disrupted digestion are *gliadorphin* from gluten and *casomorphin* from casein. As the suffix "-orphin" suggests, these amino acid chains are chemically analogous to opiate drugs like heroin and morphine, and they affect the body in ways similar to these highly addictive drugs. In fact, gliadorphin and casomorphin are called *opioid peptides*. When we consider that opiates are some of the most powerfully addictive drugs on earth, it is no wonder that dairy and carbohydrates are often staples of binge eating. This may be why members of Overeaters Anonymous who remove gluten from their diet, as the group suggests, find that their food cravings dissipate.

From brie to cheddar to feta to mozzarella, many people find cheese to be one type of food they simply cannot live without. If I recommend that patients avoid dairy products, they struggle most with giving up cheese. This is likely because cheese is a food with a particularly high concentration of casein. It takes *ten* pounds of milk to produce just *one* pound of cheese, making cheese a *highly concentrated* source of casein. For those who cannot properly digest casein, eating cheese means they are consuming a highly concentrated source of a substance they cannot metabolize. In some people, this opioid peptide in concentrated form triggers symptoms of addiction.

Specialized Digestive Enzymes

Before we take an in-depth look at how casomorphin and gliadorphin affect the body, let's first examine how these peptides are created. When a person consumes casein or gluten, the body breaks these proteins down into amino acids that are then absorbed into the bloodstream. For the intestine to digest these amino acids, the body requires a special digestive enzyme called *dipeptidyl peptidase* (DPP-IV) that is used to "snip" these peptides into individual amino acids. Some people lack adequate amounts of DPP-IV; others cannot break casein and gluten down because they consume such large quantities of casein- and gluten-containing foods that their body's supply of DPP-IV is overwhelmed. Moreover, for DPP-IV to function properly, the body needs an adequate supply of zinc.

Zinc deficiency is common in patients with a wide range of eating disorders. Women taking birth control pills are more likely to show lower zinc levels because estrogen decreases zinc absorption, increases the zinc excretion, and interferes with zinc's functioning in various parts of the body. Meat products are the main source of zinc, so those who limit or abstain from eating meat, such as vegans and vegetarians, put themselves at risk for zinc deficiency. Environmental toxins also play a role in lowering levels of zinc. The chemical Bisphenol A (BPA), found in many plastics, can also lead to zinc deficiency. Antacids contribute to zinc deficiency by decreasing absorption of zinc. Finally, strenuous exercise can promote zinc deficiency by releasing zinc into the bloodstream and body tissues, which is then excreted through sweat and, later, urine. Excessive sweating, which occurs in activities such as hot saunas and Bikram yoga, often allows trace minerals like zinc to be excreted from the body.

Regardless of the cause, an insufficiency or under-functioning of DPP-IV results in an inability to fully break down casein and gluten into amino acids. When the function of DPP-IV enzyme is compromised, casein and gluten are broken down into the larger peptides casomorphin and gliadorphin. These morphine analogs can stimulate the brain's craving and lead to dairy and gluten addiction.

It is important to note that sensitivity to casein or having high levels of casomorphin is *not* the same as lactose intolerance. This is because casein and lactose are two completely different substances. *Lactose* is a sugar in dairy products, whereas casein is a protein found in dairy products. When a person is lactose intolerant, he has too little or no *lactase*, the enzyme that breaks down lactose. Lactase does not break down casein. This means that taking Lactaid or lactase pills after eating a bowl of ice cream or a slice of cheese is not going to affect how your body breaks down casein. DPP-IV is required for this.

For more information on peptide testing, please see the *Resources* section.

Effects of Casomorphin and Gliadorphin

When casomorphin and gliadorphin enter the bloodstream, these opioid peptides travel into the brain. High blood levels of gliadorphin or casomorphin can cause addictive cravings for wheat or dairy products and alter mood in a way that complicates appetite problems.

But just as individuals have varied responses to morphine, not all people respond the same way to casomorphin and gliadorphin. For some people, eating a high volume of dairy and gluten does not cause any problems, while for others even small amounts can have detrimental effects. And for those who are affected by consumption of dairy and gluten, the effects can vary. For example, excessive amounts of gliadorphin can calm anxiety and control obsessive thoughts in some while triggering anxiety and obsessive-compulsive symptoms in others. For those who find the effects of gliadorphin and casomorphin pleasurable, products that contain gluten and casein can become impossible to resist. When the gratifying effects of casomorphin and gliadorphin wear off, individuals hooked on these substances experience withdrawals that can only be relieved once they eat that next piece of cheese or slice of cake. Withdrawal from casein and gluten, particularly heavy cheese consumption, can be just as debilitating. Patients exhibit signs of irritability, anger, anxiety, and depression, effects that mirror withdrawal from opiate drugs like heroin.

The experience of my patient Claudia serves as a dramatic example of biochemistry gone haywire through the effects of gliadorphin. When I first saw Claudia as a twenty-four-year-old college student, she revealed that since the age of sixteen, she had eaten up to four pounds of flour mixed with water each day. She couldn't remember why she had started eating flour, only that the flour paste she concocted calmed her mind and soothed her anxiety. She explained that it "tranquilized [her] racing thoughts" and that she found flour to be better than any medication she had tried.

In fact, the flour that Claudia had eaten each day for eight years functioned like a drug in her brain. Tests showed that she had very high levels of gliadorphin from incompletely digested gluten. Claudia could not stop eating flour, even for a day.

Similarly, Debbie's relationship with cheese shows just how powerful the effects of casomorphin can be. Debbie was a sixteen-year-old girl with out-of-control eating behaviors that led her family to lock the pantry door in their home because of her nighttime binge eating. She had attended multiple treatment programs as well as therapy, and had realized moderate success; however, she had also experienced a number of relapses.

When I met with Debbie, she described a history of remarkably high cheese consumption. Urinary peptide testing revealed that she had elevated casomorphin levels. I recommended that she cut casein from her diet. Debbie's withdrawal was extremely difficult. Her parents removed cheese from their home, but on a number of occasions discovered that Debbie had sneaked out of the house to obtain cheese at a friend's home or from a convenience store. Eating cheese provided her with a neurochemical "calm" similar to morphine.

Rebecca, a forty-seven-year-old woman, came to my clinic seeking treatment for binge eating disorder. She had struggled with her weight since early adolescence. Like many of my patients, she had been on multiple diets, had hired trainers for exercise programs, and had taken multiple supplement pills.

Her bingeing caused her to wake up in the middle of the night. Every evening, she binged mainly on milk and cheese, and drank "healthy" smoothies containing casein. After her casomorphin test results came back positive for high levels of this opioid peptide, she eliminated dairy and switched the protein in her milkshake to casein-free protein. Dramatically, her nighttime bingeing stopped.

If testing reveals that you have high levels of casomorphin or gliadorphin in your urine, you have found one answer to binge eating. If levels of gliadorphin are abnormally high, eliminate foods containing gluten such as bread, couscous, crackers, muffins, pasta, pretzels, and pizza. If casomorphin levels are abnormally high, eliminate foods containing casein such as baked goods, cheese, cookies, crackers, ice cream, milk, and yogurt. In both cases, you should avoid these foods for at least six months, if not permanently. Taking a DPP-IV enzyme supplement on a regular basis will aid in the digestion of any foods containing casein or gluten that you might eat unintentionally.

If you have high levels of gliadorphin and casomorphin in your urine, you will probably find it difficult to avoid eating foods with gluten and casein because of their morphine-like effects on body and mind. You may even experience withdrawal symptoms similar to those from other opiates, including irritability, tremors, cravings, or sweating. To help address these uncomfortable symptoms, you need to taper off gluten and dairy slowly, particularly if cheese is your "drug of choice." Medications can also lessen the discomfort associated with withdrawal and will be discussed in more detail in Chapter 11.

Please see the *Resources* section for information on how to obtain DPP-IV supplements.

Testing for Elevated Levels of Casomorphin and Gliadorphin

It is important to test for elevated levels of casomorphin and gliadorphin *before* you eliminate foods containing these proteins. I do not advocate excluding gluten and casein from your diet unless you have celiac disease, food allergies, or excess amounts of opioid peptides. Unnecessarily removing major food groups from your diet can cause deficiencies of vitamins and minerals that can lead to health problems.

The opiate peptide test is a first-morning-urine test that can be completed at home and sent to a laboratory to be analyzed. Though it is not always covered by insurance, the cost of the test ranges between $100 and $300.

Eliminating foods that may fuel an addictive process—excessive sugar, as well as wheat and dairy if your tests reveal sensitivities to gluten and casein—is a fundamental answer to appetite control. Remember that binge eating and food addiction are biologically-based problems and therefore require biologically-based solutions. Enjoying the New Hope involves *not* taking substances into your body that perpetuate disordered appetite and trap you on a frantic roller-coaster ride.

Summary

It isn't a coincidence that, during a binge, people often crave foods such as bread, cheese, ice cream, cookies, and crackers. Grain and dairy products contain specific proteins, called gluten and casein, respectively, which can be highly addictive when not digested properly. Gluten and casein must be broken down into tiny peptides before they can be utilized by the body to build important hormones and neurotransmitters. In some individuals, however, these proteins are not fully broken down and instead remain as bulkier peptides called gliadorphin and casomorphin. These larger protein derivatives are called opioid peptides, as they are highly addictive and chemically similar to drugs such as heroin and morphine.

Complications with gluten metabolism are also noted in celiac disease, a chronic autoimmune condition. In individuals with celiac disease, the body perpetually mistakes gluten for a foreign invader and rallies to launch damaging attacks. Ultimately, these confused immune reactions result in severe digestive distress, inflammation, and nutrient deficiencies, as well as increase the risk of cancer and other health problems.

Foods containing gluten and casein aren't unequivocally evil. In fact, for those able to tolerate them, grain and dairy products bolster health. However, in sensitive individuals these tasty foods provoke harmful physiological, psychological, and emotional reactions. Nutritional testing can direct you to make appropriate dietary shifts that will support your individual biochemistry while minimizing the risk of nutrient discrepancies and other complications. If you test positive for sensitivity to these two peptides, I recommend eliminating casein- and gluten-containing foods to minimize symptoms of withdrawal such as irritability, tremors, cravings, or sweating.

Key Points

- Gluten is a protein found in many grain-based foods such as bread, pasta, crackers, cookies, pastries, and cake. Casein is a protein found in all dairy products including milk, cheese, and yogurt.
- Once ingested, gluten and casein are broken down into tiny peptides that are used by the body to create hormones and neurotransmitters, which are essential to health.
- In some people, gluten and casein are not fully digested and instead remain as larger peptides called gliadorphin and casomorphin.
- The incompletely broken-down gliadorphin and casomorphin are opioid peptides, highly addictive substances that are chemically similar to drugs such as heroin and morphine.
- Some people are not affected by the consumption of gluten and casein because they are able to properly break them down. For others, however, eating gluten- or casein-rich foods can have damaging physical, psychological, and emotional effects.
- Celiac disease is a specific condition in which the immune system confuses gluten for a foreign invader, and mistakenly launches an attack. These autoimmune reactions are both energy-consuming and damaging, and can result in severe digestive problems, inflammation, nutrient deficiencies, and an increased risk of chronic illness.
- Individualized vitamin and mineral supplementation is a crucial component of effective eating disorder treatment.
- Cheese is a highly concentrated source of casein; as such it can be a problematic and addictive food for those who cannot properly digest it.
- The body requires a special enzyme called dipeptidyl peptidase, or DPP-IV, to break gluten and casein down into smaller peptides. Some people lack enough DPP-IV, either because supplies have been depleted by overconsuming gluten- and casein-rich foods or due to a lack of the necessary nutritional building blocks.
- A common reason for inadequate levels of DPP-IV is a deficiency of the vitamin zinc. Zinc deficiency can be caused by many factors

- such as lack of meat in the diet, over-exercise, antacid usage, or exposure to environmental toxins like BPA.
- Casein- and gluten-containing foods have beneficial nutrient profiles when well-tolerated. Proper nutritional testing must be done prior to making diet changes in order to reduce the risk of nutrient discrepancies.
- If necessary, the elimination of casein- or gluten-containing foods should be done gradually so as to minimize withdrawal symptoms, which may include irritability, tremors, and cravings.

PART II.
PERSONALIZED NUTRITIONAL SUPPLEMENTS FOR BINGE EATING AND FOOD ADDICTION

8
LABORATORY EVALUATIONS FOR INDIVIDUALIZED NUTRITIONAL SUPPORT

As binge eating and food addiction are biologically-based problems, effective solutions must necessarily begin with biology. Restoring a healthy appetite starts with determining your unique biochemistry. Based on results from your laboratory evaluations, you can begin a program of nutritional support tailored just for you. Traditionally, the evaluation of nutritional status has not been a part of a psychiatric examination. After treating thousands of patients with binge eating disorder and other disordered eating patterns, I believe a comprehensive metabolic evaluation is a critical component of helping a person regain control over his or her appetite. Results from laboratory assessments are used as a basis for developing a personalized nutritional program that optimizes health, enhances long-term recovery and, most importantly, prevents relapse.

A metabolic assessment provides the answer to an often-neglected question: are there any biological factors contributing to or actually causing your tendency to binge and lose control of your appetite? The answer is often "Yes!"

Most nutritional deficiencies are not discernable from a standard physical or psychiatric examination. A nutritional assessment for disordered eating involves a number of laboratory tests. Some are conventional and commonly performed in a doctor's office; others are not as well-known. Discovering nutritional deficiencies and correcting them through proper supplementation will help you participate more effectively in your own recovery, find your way off the roller-coaster ride, and discover the New Hope.

Getting Started

I recommend the following tests, which can be ordered by any physician:

- Amino acids
- Complete blood count (CBC) with differential
- Celiac disease screening (anti-tissue transglutaminase antibody and anti-gliadin antibody tests)
- Coenzyme Q10
- C-reactive protein (CRP)
- Lipid panel, cholesterol HDL/LDL triglycerides
- Comprehensive chemistry panel
- Copper level
- Cortisol: adrenal stress test
- DHEA-S
- Estrogen and progesterone
- Essential fatty acids
- Folate
- Food allergies
- Homocysteine
- Iron and ferritin
- Magnesium
- Methylmalonic acid
- Trace minerals
- Thyroid function test
- Uric acid
- Urinary organic acids
- Urinary peptides casomorphin and gliadorphin
- Vitamin B12
- Vitamin D
- Zinc

Additional testing may be recommended based on symptoms and results of initial screening labs.

Amino Acids

Neurotransmitters, like all proteins, are created from amino acids. The majority of these are obtained through dietary sources. Serotonin, the "master appetite controller," is manufactured from the amino acid tryptophan, while dopamine and norepinephrine come from the amino acid phenylalanine. Tryptophan and phenylalanine, along with many other amino acids, are thus essential neurotransmitter *precursors* – molecules or compounds that participate in chemical reactions that produce other compounds.

When these amino acid precursors are in short supply in your brain, levels of corresponding neurotransmitters may also be low, which can lead to appetite problems. Too little tryptophan can result in low levels of serotonin. This can lead to depression and bingeing on carbohydrates. Too little phenylalanine or tyrosine can cause lowered dopamine levels, triggering fatigue and difficulty concentrating. Too little norepinephrine can cause depression, which can manifest as either an abnormally increased or decreased appetite.

Although not a routine test for most physicians, *serum amino acid testing* has been one of the most valuable tests I recommend. All the peptides, neurotransmitters, and hormones involved in appetite and satiety are produced from amino acids obtained from one's diet. If there is a deficiency of amino acids, disordered eating patterns are common.

Complete Blood Count (CBC) with Differential

The CBC measures white blood cell count and types (called differential), red blood cell count and characteristics, hemoglobin, hematocrit, and platelets. Anemia, which can lead to depression, is indicated by low red blood cell count, low hemoglobin, and low hematocrit. Certain characteristics of the red blood cell, designated MCH, MCV, or MCHC, can pinpoint the nutrient deficiency causing the anemia, whether it is copper, folate, iron, or vitamin B12.

White blood cells can be abnormally high from an infection, an allergic reaction, or leukemia, or abnormally low due to medication reactions or low levels of zinc. Platelets play a role in blood clotting, and both high and low levels are abnormal. Low levels can cause excessive bleeding and bruising.

Celiac Screening

Celiac disease is a sensitivity to the protein gluten found in wheat and other grains. If you have celiac disease, your body mistakenly identifies gluten as a foreign invader and launches an immune attack. Celiac disease results in the destruction of intestinal *villi*, the hair-like projections lining the intestine, which impairs the absorption of nutrients. Deficiencies of essential amino acids, vitamins, and trace minerals are common in patients suffering from celiac disease. These deficiencies result in neuropeptide and neurotransmitter imbalances, and often lead to disordered eating behavior. Scientific research has demonstrated that people with celiac disease have higher rates of anxiety and depression as compared to the general population.

Research has shown that individuals who adopt a gluten-free diet are at an increased risk for disordered eating. People with celiac disease have to be vigilant about what they eat. Preoccupation with the avoidance of certain foods can develop into an unhealthy obsession. New research supports our understanding of how the activation of the inflammatory response in celiac disease can trigger symptoms of depression and an eating disorder.

Screening for celiac disease involves examining a blood sample to determine the presence of two antibodies that the body manufactures in response to gluten: *anti-tissue transglutaminase* and *anti-gliadin*. To confirm a positive result, a biopsy of the small intestine can be performed. An endoscope is inserted down the throat, through the stomach, and into the small intestine. Tissue samples taken from its lining are examined under a microscope to identify characteristic changes seen in celiac disease, including shrunken, flattened villi.

Lipid Panel

A lipid panel measures the levels of cholesterol, triglycerides, high-density lipoprotein (HDL), and low-density lipoprotein (LDL) through a blood test. Recent studies suggest that low total cholesterol levels are associated with depression, as well as with suicidal thoughts and behavior. Scientists have theorized that low levels of cholesterol result in lowered production of serotonin and inefficient functioning of serotonin receptors in the brain. Cholesterol is the precursor molecule for all steroid hormones, including cortisol, testosterone, estrogen, and progesterone. Low cholesterol has been implicated in many physical and mental health issues. A disorder of cholesterol metabolism, either because it is high or low, plays a role in disordered eating.

Comprehensive Chemistry Panel

This group of blood tests is used to evaluate organ function and to provide a preliminary check for diabetes, liver disease, and kidney problems. The test results include important information about electrolyte status, acid-base balance, kidney function, liver function, blood sugar, and protein levels. This panel can also assess a person's zinc status by measuring *alkaline phosphatase*, an enzyme produced in the presence of zinc. A low alkaline phosphatase level is an indicator of a functional zinc deficiency.

Copper

Low copper levels can lead to symptoms of depression, which is unsurprising considering that copper is required for the synthesis of the neurotransmitters norepinephrine and dopamine. A deficiency of a form of copper called *ceruloplasmin* can cause anemia, which itself can precipitate depressive symptoms. On the other hand, abnormally high levels of copper can be associated with psychological symptoms such as aggression, paranoia, and anxiety. Copper levels are determined by blood tests and by hair testing. Levels that are abnormal may be treated with supplementation or modification to the diet.

Coenzyme Q10

CoQ10, or *coenzyme Q10*, is composed of a group of electron carriers that collectively generate energy in the form of ATP (adenosine triphosphate). It is not considered an essential nutrient, which means our bodies are capable of manufacturing this enzyme on their own. However, the most readily available dietary sources of CoQ10 are foods such as meat, poultry, fish, nuts and soybean oils. Deficiencies of CoQ10 usually present with compromised nerve and muscle functioning. CoQ10 deficiencies can also lead to depression, which in turn may lead to eating disturbances and appetite problems.

Cortisol

Cortisol, known as the stress hormone, is involved in appetite regulation. The adrenal glands are responsible for your responses to stress; accordingly, the measurement of adrenal hormones such as cortisol can be a reliable indicator of your adrenal function and how your body deals with stress. Abnormal levels of cortisol have been reported in women with anorexia nervosa as well as in those with obesity. High levels of cortisol have been observed in women with disordered eating behavior, suggesting that abnormalities in appetite regulation are associated with eating disorder pathology.

Cortisol can also stimulate intense cravings for sugar and tends to make cells resistant to insulin. This in turn increases the stimulation of fat deposits in your body and leads you on a vicious cycle of bingeing on sugar-laden foods, which triggers the cascade of disordered eating.

Cortisol levels can be measured through a blood or saliva test. Cortisol levels throughout the day may be measured by analyzing your saliva. Test results can reveal biochemical imbalances that contribute to chronic stress and adrenal fatigue, impairing your ability to regulate appetite.

C-Reactive Protein (CRP)

C-reactive protein (CRP) is a protein that is produced by the liver. The presence of an elevated CRP level indicates that there is inflammation present in the body. Elevated CRP levels may also be due to a lack of sleep, stress, excessive exercise, infections, overeating, and obesity. Chronic inflammation can lead to a higher risk of cardiovascular disease, diabetes, and depression. Studies have demonstrated that individuals with elevated CRP levels have a higher risk for developing depression. The majority of patients we see for binge eating have increased CRP levels. Several studies suggest that lifestyle changes, such as regular exercise in overweight individuals, have been able to decrease CRP levels and stimulate weight loss. C-reactive protein levels may be measured by a blood test.

DHEA-S

Dehydroepiandrosterone (DHEA), the most common steroid hormone in the body, is the "raw material" used to produce the sex hormones testosterone and estrogen and up to one hundred and fifty other steroid hormones. DHEA helps the body burn calories and fat at a rapid pace and store glucose. With age, metabolism slows and the body starts to burn fewer calories; by the mid-thirties, most of the hormones that keep metabolism going at a speedy rate are on the downslide. Production of DHEA is at its peak in your mid-twenties, after which it drops precipitously, falling about ninety percent between the ages of twenty and ninety. Age-related weight gain and abdominal obesity are believed to be at least partially due to this drop in DHEA.

Studies have shown that DHEA has a wide range of anti-obesity effects. It stimulates the resting metabolic rate, increases fat burning, and decreases caloric intake, resulting in reductions in body weight, total body fat, and abdominal fat. DHEA also has an insulin-like effect, aiding in the disposal of excess glucose. A study of fifty-six people ages sixty-five to seventy-eight who had age-related DHEA decreases found that daily doses of 50 milligrams of DHEA for six months caused significant decreases in participants' subcutaneous (under the skin) and abdominal fat, as well as significant increases in insulin sensitivity. Animal studies indicate that DHEA helps direct the body to burn body fat rather than body protein.

Side effects of taking DHEA supplements can include acne, excess facial hair in women and, at high doses or with long-term use, an increased risk of developing certain hormone-related cancers. All of these side effects are primarily due to the conversion of DHEA to testosterone and estrogen. However, they are not seen with a metabolic by-product of DHEA called 3-acetyl-7-oxo-dehydroepiandrosterone (7-Keto). In one study, two groups of volunteers followed weight-loss diets and exercised regularly. One group also received 100 milligrams of 7-Keto twice daily, while the other received a placebo. By the end of the study, those taking 7-Keto had lost three times as much weight as those taking the placebo.

Adequate DHEA-S levels can be assessed through a simple blood test. If blood levels are optimal, then supplementation is not likely to be beneficial. If the blood test reflects low DHEA-S levels, I recommend supplementation to normalize DHEA-S levels. DHEA-S levels should be monitored every three months.

Estrogen and Progesterone

Estrogen and *progesterone* are secreted by the ovaries under the control of the hypothalamus and the pituitary gland. There's no doubt that the female hormones estrogen and progesterone influence mood: Many women can sense the changes as they move through their menstrual cycle and again as they approach and go through menopause. Hormonal influences on mood in women are much more complex than they are in men, and there is no simple formula that titrates estrogen to prevent depression. Instead, the key is to balance hormone levels, a tricky process that should be done only under the supervision of an endocrinologist.

Many women report that they experience an increase in food cravings, particularly for carbohydrates, sugar, and salt, when their menstrual cycle draws near. A link between estrogen, progesterone, and food cravings was established in a recent study conducted by the University of Texas Southwestern Medical Center. Researchers found that estrogen regulates energy expenditure, appetite, and body weight. Insufficient estrogen receptors in certain parts of the brain may lead to obesity and an increased risk of cardiovascular disease. In this study, female mice lacking a certain estrogen receptor became overweight and developed diabetes and heart disease. These results may shed light on the fact that women may have more food cravings when menstruation is about to occur, as estrogen and progesterone levels are then at their lowest.

Considerable controversy surrounds the issue of *hormone replacement therapy* for women. Conventional hormone replacement therapy with synthetic hormones was the standard of care until studies conducted by the Women's Health Initiative, a fifteen-year-long research program involving forty medical centers and over one hundred and sixty thousand women across the country, received national attention. The Women's Health Initiative was launched to address health concerns in postmenopausal women. Most notable was its study of estrogen plus progestin hormone therapy in postmenopausal women. The study was abruptly ended three years early when the clinicians involved concluded that the risks of the therapy outweighed the benefits. Women receiving the combination hormone therapy experienced increased risks of invasive breast cancer, coronary heart disease, stroke, and pulmonary embolism when compared to women taking only placebo pills.

Due to these concerns, many physicians have consistently found natural, bio-identical hormones preferable to synthetic ones. Although few research studies have been conducted that support the benefits of natural hormones, the potential side effects of synthetic hormones far outweigh the benefits. Like all nutritional or natural therapies, further research on natural and bio-identical hormone therapy is unlikely, as this type of treatment is not patentable and therefore will not generate large profits for pharmaceutical companies. Make sure you work with a practitioner who is experienced in the use of natural or bio-identical hormones before initiating any type of hormone replacement therapy.

Essential Fatty Acids

Essential fatty acids (EFA) are the building blocks of every cell membrane in the human body. Necessary for critical biological processes in the body, they are called "essential" because your body can't manufacture them; they must, therefore, be obtained from the diet. *Omega-3 fatty acids* come primarily from fish or fish oil, while *omega-6 fatty acids* are obtained through vegetable oils and grains. All essential fatty acids play crucial roles in brain and nerve function, normal growth and development, and the regulation of inflammation. Dietary fat restriction can often result in essential fatty acid deficiencies and increase the risk of developing mental health problems such as ADHD, anxiety, and depression.

Populations that routinely consume high levels of omega-3s in the form of fish or fish oil have lower incidence and prevalence rates of depression, while those consuming low levels display increased depression rates. Numerous studies have shown that omega-3 supplements can be helpful in treating depression, ADHD, and anxiety, all of which are associated with binge eating and obesity. Omega-3 deficiencies have also been associated with an increased incidence of suicide.

Abnormally high or low levels of various fatty acids can be treated with supplementation or through dietary modification.

Folate

If you're tired, depressed, anxious, or struggling with fatigue, it could be due to low levels of *folate* (also known as *folic acid*). Folate levels may be checked by a simple blood test.

Folate is necessary for red blood cell formation, normal psychological function, tissue and cellular repair, and DNA production. Low levels can produce a condition called *macrocytic anemia*, in which the body produces larger but fewer red blood cells that have a decreased ability to carry oxygen, resulting in fatigue.

Too little folate, which is used to produce neurotransmitters, can contribute to depression and can underlie many other psychological and neurological problems including anxiety, confusion, hallucinations, dementia, and numbness and tingling of the hands and feet.

Folate must be converted into *L-methylfolate* in order to cross the blood-brain barrier and be made available for neurotransmitter synthesis. People with genetic mutations called *methlentetrahydrofolate reductase* (MTHFR) *polymorphisms* have impaired folate metabolism. Several studies show that people with variants of the MTHFR gene have a higher incidence of depression and require higher levels of folate supplementation. Genetic testing to check whether you have MTHFR polymorphisms can be invaluable in in the treatment of coexisting depression and eating disorders.

Folate supplementation will be discussed in more detail in Chapter 10.

Food Allergies

Allergies are the result of an immune system that has gone haywire. As if out of the blue, the immune system begins to identify normal, harmless substances (*allergens*) as foreign invaders and to send immune system cells (*antibodies*) on a mission to wipe them out. This starts an unnecessary war within the body that can damage cells, tissues, organs, and even entire organ systems. Allergies stemming from ingested foods cause obvious symptoms such as stomach pain, nausea, vomiting, and diarrhea, but can also contribute to food cravings, depression, and anxiety.

RAST (Radio-Allergo-Sobertent Test) testing evaluates *IgE* (immunoglobulin E) *medical allergies*. This is the common allergy test that is performed in a physician's office to detect immediate hypersensitivities to foods such as peanuts and shellfish. IgE allergies may trigger severe reactions that can cause anaphylactic shock, resulting in a significant drop in blood pressure, rapid heart rate, airway constriction, and loss of consciousness.

IgG-mediated food sensitivities are another type of food allergy. The reactions they trigger are known as *delayed hypersensitivity reactions*. Symptoms may occur hours or even days after ingestion and are commonly associated with mood and behavior changes as well as an increase in food cravings. Often, patients crave the very foods to which they have IgG sensitivities. IgG testing is completed through a blood test that can identify problem foods to avoid. In many cases, moods improve and cravings disappear once the foods are eliminated from the diet.

Homocysteine

Homocysteine, an amino acid produced by the body, is normally converted quickly to another amino acid called cysteine with the help of folate and vitamins B6 and B12. Research shows that high homocysteine levels are associated with depression. Although not all depressed people have elevated homocysteine and not all people with elevated homocysteine levels are depressed, data from the Health in Men Study involving 3,762 men found that higher levels of homocysteine increased depression risk.

Although an abnormally high level of homocysteine is not directly related to appetite changes, it can be viewed as an early warning sign of nutrient deficiencies that do play a role in regulating appetite, including folate and vitamins B6 and B12.

Iron and Ferritin

Iron is needed by the body to create *hemoglobin*, the oxygen-carrying protein found in red blood cells. A lack of iron can cause *iron-deficiency anemia*, a condition in which the red blood cells can't deliver enough oxygen to the rest of the body. Women who are menstruating or pregnant, new mothers, vegetarians, dieters, people with anorexia, and patients with celiac disease are all at high risk of developing iron-deficiency anemia and its classic symptoms of fatigue.

The fatigue associated with iron-deficiency anemia often contributes to cravings for sugar and more calories. Iron-deficiency anemia may be hard to diagnose during the early stages since blood levels can at first appear normal. Checking levels of *ferritin*, which is the protein carrier for iron, is the best way of detecting an iron deficiency.

Magnesium

The mineral magnesium is found in every cell in the body, with more than half of the body's store residing in the bones. It is sometimes thought of as the "opposite" of calcium because it helps to balance calcium's actions: calcium, for example, constricts and contracts blood vessels, while magnesium relaxes and widens them. Magnesium is necessary for heart function, neurotransmitter synthesis, the removal of toxic substances, and the conversion of protein, fat and carbohydrates into energy. Stress increases the excretion of magnesium, making magnesium deficiency more likely.

Poor intake or increased magnesium excretion can lead to depression, anxiety, insomnia, difficulty concentrating, nausea, and weakness, all of which can alter your appetite. Magnesium deficiency is common in patients with binge eating disorder.

Thyroid

Thyroid hormones play a role in circadian rhythms and are responsible for regulating the rate at which the body uses energy. The thyroid gland takes up iodine and converts it into the thyroid hormones *thyroxine* (T4) and *triiodothyronine* (T3). When concentrations of these hormones drop too low, the pituitary gland releases *thyroid-stimulating hormone* (TSH), which prompts the thyroid gland to produce more. When levels normalize, the thyroid stops producing these hormones.

A thyroid panel is a group of tests that measures the amount of TSH, T4 and T3 in your blood. Too little T4 and T3 causes *hypothyroidism*, a condition that lowers the metabolic rate and increases the tendency toward weight gain, loss of appetite, fatigue, constipation, cold intolerance and menstrual irregularities. On the other hand, too much T4 and T3 causes *hyperthyroidism*, which steps up the metabolic rate and causes weight loss, an increased heart rate, anxiety, insomnia, weakness and, again, a loss of appetite.

Low thyroid hormones promote weight gain, which can increase a tendency toward disordered eating and contribute to depression, anxiety, and other psychological problems. Because one of the symptoms of low thyroid can be a *loss* of appetite, it's possible that a person with hypothyroidism may eat very little yet still gain weight. Screening for thyroid problems is an important step in diagnosing and treating disordered eating. Levels of thyroid hormones can be assessed through a simple blood test.

Urinary Organic Acids

Abnormally high levels of *organic acids* result from the blockage of one or more of the body's metabolic pathways, which prompts excretion of acids through the urine. Organic acids in the urine reveal the functioning of multiple biological processes, including neurotransmitter function, detoxification, digestive imbalances, energy production, and nutrient deficiencies.

Urinary organic acids act as markers for the depletion of nutrients at the cellular level. For example, one indication of a vitamin B6 deficiency is excessive amounts of an organic acid called *kynurenate* in the urine. Vitamin B6 plays a key role in synthesis of all major neurotransmitters.

HPHPA, or *3-(3-hydroxyphenyl)-3-hydroxypropionic acid*, is an abnormal metabolite produced by gastrointestinal bacteria of the *Clostridia* species and is elevated in many psychiatric conditions. HPHPA is frequently associated with behavioral and neurological problems, such as ADHD, depression, OCD, and psychosis. Yeast metabolites can be detected in the organic acid test. Yeast thrives on sugar, and an overgrowth of yeast stimulates the appetite for foods containing refined sugars and carbohydrates. As a result, insulin levels increase, metabolism slows down, and fatigue and food cravings follow. This triggers the vicious cycle of disordered appetite, as you reach for sugar-laden foods to acquire a boost of energy to compensate for your fatigue.

Overgrowth of yeast occurs most often after taking antibiotics that reduce the number of beneficial bacteria in your body. Poor nutrition and environmental stress are other factors that can contribute to yeast overgrowth. In many cases, high levels of HPHPA or an overgrowth of yeast can be controlled by supplementation with high-dose probiotics. The urinary organic acid test is performed using a sample of first morning urine. The presence and levels of up to seventy different compounds can be tested using one sample.

Urinary Peptides

The opiate peptides *casomorphin* and *gliadorphin* appear in the urine when the naturally occurring proteins casein (found in milk) and gluten (found in wheat, rye, barley and other grains) are not completely digested, wreaking havoc by building up to unhealthy levels.

When properly digested, casomorphin and gliadorphin are broken into small protein fragments and safely absorbed into the bloodstream.

Problems in breakdown occur because the protease enzyme called *dipeptidyl peptidase* (DPP-IV) is insufficient or inactive.

High levels of gliadorphin or casomorphin can cause addictive cravings for wheat or dairy products, as well as mood-altering effects that complicate appetite problems (as discussed in detail in Chapter 7). The presence of gliadorphin or casomorphin is identified through a urinary peptide test. High levels of either peptide in the urine usually indicate that the DPP-IV enzyme is either ineffective or in short supply. If levels of gliadorphin are abnormally high, foods containing gluten such as bread, couscous, crackers, muffins, pasta, pretzels, and pizza, should be eliminated from the diet. If casomorphin levels are abnormally high, foods containing casein should be eliminated, including baked goods, cheese, ice cream, milk, and yogurt. In both cases, it is helpful to take a DPP-IV enzyme supplement on a regular basis to assist with proper digestion.

Vitamin B12

Vitamin B12 is crucial to the manufacture and growth of red blood cells, the production of DNA, and the maintenance of a healthy central nervous system. A vitamin B12 deficiency can cause pernicious anemia (a decrease in red blood cells), damage to the white matter of the spinal cord and brain, and numbness and tingling in the hands and feet. It can also produce psychiatric symptoms including fatigue, depression, anxiety, memory loss, paranoia, and behavioral changes.

Vitamin B12 deficiency can result from poor dietary intake or poor absorption of the vitamin. It's frequently observed in vegetarians, vegans, or others who restrict their intake of animal products, since B12 is found only in foods of animal origin. Poor absorption of B12 is usually caused by a lack of the protein *intrinsic factor*, a common condition in the elderly. Intrinsic factor combines with B12 in the stomach to form a complex, which then travels to the end of the small intestine where it is absorbed. If vitamin B12 is not bound to intrinsic factor, it simply passes through the intestines unabsorbed.

A B12 deficiency, often seen in individuals with anxiety and depression, can promote eating disorders and appetite problems. Several epidemiological studies have shown a higher prevalence of depression in those with low blood levels of B12. Conversely, higher levels of B12 are associated with better long-term outcomes in depression.

Vitamin C

Vitamin C is an important antioxidant responsible for maintaining general health. Our evolutionary ancestors lost the ability to synthesize vitamin C long ago, and thus we must obtain it through diet. There is evidence that vitamin C can counter the effects of fructose in causing metabolic syndrome or insulin resistance. Individuals with metabolic syndrome and diabetes often exhibit deficiencies in vitamin C.

Vitamin C was recently found helpful in treating depression. A study published in *Nutrition Journal* revealed that vitamin C may be a promising adjunct to antidepressant therapy. A group of patients given the antidepressant fluoxetine (Prozac) plus 1,000 milligrams per day of vitamin C showed a significant decrease in depressive symptoms compared to a group that took fluoxetine plus a placebo.

Vitamin D

It is *essential* to evaluate vitamin D in all patients with appetite problems, weight problems, or disordered eating. A vitamin D deficiency is impossible to identify without testing serum blood levels. Vitamin D is often called the sunshine vitamin since it can be synthesized by your body when you are exposed to the sun's ultraviolet rays. It is an essential nutrient involved in a wide variety of biochemical processes throughout the body, including the regulation of appetite. Specifically, vitamin D regulates the synthesis of the neurotransmitter serotonin; serotonin, in addition to its powerful effects on mood and cognition, is thought to play a role in appetite regulation and satiety. Put another way, vitamin D helps to manufacture a chemical which can boost feelings of fullness and hunger satisfaction.

Supplementation of vitamin D is based on your lab values. I typically recommend between 5,000 or 10,000 IU until you have a sustained vitamin D blood level of approximately 50 ng/ml. A substantial body of scientific evidence demonstrates an association between low vitamin D levels and depressive illness. Research has shown that vitamin D deficiency is significantly correlated with depression risk, as well as with increased rates of depressive disorders around the globe. Although environmental factors such as nutrition and sun exposure are major determinants of vitamin D status, genetics are also responsible for a portion of the variance found in blood levels. Testing vitamin D levels is the only way to determine if vitamin D supplementation is required.

Zinc

Zinc, an essential nutrient for all living organisms, is found in every cell and tissue in the human body. It affects biological processes ranging from DNA synthesis to cell renewal and is a crucial component of over two hundred enzymes, including all the major gastrointestinal enzymes. Zinc also plays an important role in immune system function, wound healing, and growth.

Low levels of zinc have been correlated with depression and eating disorders. Zinc deficiency diminishes the senses of taste and smell, decreases appetite, and causes nausea. Too little zinc also contributes to mood disturbances and psychological problems, including anxiety, depression, lethargy, and impaired concentration. At least half of people with anorexia have measurable zinc deficiencies and an impaired capacity to absorb zinc from foods and supplements.

Blood tests measuring zinc levels are not always reliable, as they may register normal results until a deficiency has become severe. The best method for measuring zinc status is the *zinc taste test*. Developed in the 1980s by Dr. Derek Bryce-Smith, it involves giving an individual a taste of zinc sulfate solution and observing his or her response. The response is measured based on a scale. People who are zinc-deficient note either no taste (a Category 1 on the scale) or very little taste (Category 2). A bitter or metallic taste is indicative of an adequate zinc level (Category 3 for milk taste versus a Category 4 for stronger taste). This test can identify even subtle deficiencies and may be useful in revealing factors that may contribute to disordered eating.

Other Issues

Recent headlines in the national press have claimed that multivitamins are worthless. The notion that multivitamins improve cognitive function and prevent cardiovascular disease and cancer were debunked. Reports from major news agencies such as *The New York Times* and *The Wall Street Journal* described recently-published scientific papers. In December 2013, the *Annals of Journal Medicine* published a literature review examining several trials and studies on multivitamin supplements which together included over four hundred thousand participants. After reviewing the available evidence, the authors of the literature review concluded that there was no clear evidence of a beneficial effect of supplements on various health issues. These recent studies are highly controversial as they were poorly controlled and did not utilize high-quality supplements. However, the results do reflect important information about health and biochemical individuality. Multivitamins are *not* magic bullets. Taking multivitamin supplements without individualized laboratory testing is not always helpful.

Understanding the root of your problem is the first step toward reclaiming a healthy appetite. The tests described above provide the comprehensive metabolic evaluation you need to uncover any physical or nutritional deficiencies that may be contributing to your issues with appetite. From this metabolic profile, you and your healthcare provider can create an individualized treatment program based on your unique biochemistry.

James Greenblatt, MD

Summary

Few psychiatrists utilize lab testing to assess health in the treatment of eating disorders. However, a metabolic assessment provides invaluable insight as to any biological factors that may be contributing to appetite problems. Information obtained from a metabolic assessment can allow us to target nutritional and metabolic imbalances that are interfering with the body's appetite-regulation mechanisms, as opposed to merely treating the symptoms of such imbalances. Disordered eating is infrequently caused by a deficiency of just one nutrient; instead, it is more commonly the result of a combination of deficiencies and imbalances. Identifying nutritional deficiencies and correcting them with proper supplementation will support recovery from a disordered appetite.

Laboratory testing is the foundation of a personalized nutritional approach. Your individual biochemistry is as unique as your thumbprint. Laboratory testing results will help tailor a treatment plan designed for your unique biochemistry.

Key Points

Laboratory testing for binge eating and food addiction includes:

- Amino acids
- Complete Blood Count (CBC) with differential
- Celiac disease screening
- CoQ10 Enzyme
- C-Reactive Protein (CRP)
- Lipid panel, cholesterol HDL/LDL triglycerides
- Comprehensive Chemistry Panel
- Copper level
- Cortisol: Adrenal Stress Test
- DHEA-S
- Estrogen and progesterone

- Essential fatty acids
- Folate and vitamin B12
- Food allergies
- Homocysteine
- Iron and ferritin
- Magnesium
- Methylmalonic acid
- Trace minerals
- Thyroid function test
- Uric Acid
- Urinary organic acids
- Urinary peptides
- Vitamin B12

Additional testing may be recommended based on symptoms and results of initial screening labs.

9
CONTROLLING APPETITE WITH AMINO ACID SUPPLEMENTS

You should be relieved to learn that appetite control does not have to entail a lifelong battle. You can give up slavish counting of calories and the daily rituals and resolutions to be more self-disciplined. Since disordered eating is often related to biochemical imbalances, the solution must incorporate biochemical interventions. To control appetite, you need to experience a sense of fullness rather than a continuous craving for more. Amino acids can do just that.

Amino acids are organic compounds that combine in various ways to make proteins. The amino acids form the molecular basis for neurotransmitters and neuropeptides, the keys to appetite control in the human body.

Supporting the diet with amino acids is the first step toward controlling appetite. Many patients experience a dramatic decline in cravings and in the desire to binge soon after they begin taking amino acid supplements. In my thirty years of clinical practice, I've found amino acids especially helpful in cases of binge eating, chronic cravings, depression, and anxiety. In fact, I will go so far as to say that supplemental amino acids are the most helpful intervention that I've found in treating these illnesses.

The amino acids are the building blocks of proteins. Along with carbohydrates and fats, proteins are the raw materials we take into our bodies. While carbohydrates and fats are simply structured, the proteins are more complicated. Amino acid molecules, which contain carbon, hydrogen, oxygen, and nitrogen atoms in specific configurations, are strung together in unique sequences called *peptides*, which then combine to form proteins. Our bodies manufacture more than fifty thousand different proteins. All of these are comprised of different combinations of just twenty amino acids.

Essential and Nonessential Amino Acids

The twenty amino acids are classified as either "essential" or "nonessential." The liver manufactures eleven of these twenty amino acids, while the remaining nine must be obtained through the diet. These category names are actually somewhat misleading. *All* the amino acids are essential to health; it's just that nine of them must be obtained from outside the body, either from food or from supplements. If these nine are supplied in adequate quantities, the body can manufacture the other eleven.

Amino Acids

Nonessential	Essential
Alanine	Histidine (in infants)
Arginine	Isoleucine
Asparagine	Leucine
Aspartate	Lysine
Carnitine	Methionine
Cysteine	Phenylalanine
Glutamate	Threonine
Glutamine	Tryptophan
Glycine	Valine
Histidine	
Proline	

Nonessential	Essential
Serine	
Taurine	
Tyrosine	

How the Amino Acids Work

Once amino acids are ingested into the body, they enter the digestive tract, where they are stripped from the protein molecules. Then they are distributed as raw materials that, along with enzymes, vitamins, and minerals, spark the chemical reactions that keep our bodies functioning. The metabolic pathways formed by amino acids build and repair muscle tissue and produce enzymes and hormones. In fact, they have thousands of functions within the body. Many of these involve appetite regulation.

Our thoughts, emotions and behaviors are influenced and regulated by neurotransmitters and neuropeptides. These chemical messengers relay information from one nerve cell to another throughout the brain. As neurotransmitters are released from nerve cells, the resulting electrical impulses affect how we think, feel, and act. Amino acid levels that are too low can result in abnormally low neurotransmitter and neuropeptide levels. When levels of the neurotransmitters serotonin, dopamine, and norepinephrine are low, appetite disturbances and eating problems can develop. In fact, all psychiatric medications affect the functioning of neurotransmitters and neuropeptides.

Neuropeptides

The *neuropeptides* are small molecules used by neurons to communicate with each other. The many neuropeptides in the human body have a wide range of brain functions; some play critical roles in appetite and appetite control.

The neuropeptides are now the focus of the most promising research in appetite and obesity, because all the triggers of hunger and satiety within our bodies can be traced to them. Ghrelin, neuropeptide Y, and the opioid peptides stimulate hunger, while leptin and cholecystokinin (CCK) decrease hunger and induce the feeling of satiety.

When your stomach is empty, cells in its lining produce the peptide *ghrelin*, which increases hunger. Ghrelin is a peptide made up of twenty-eight amino acids, and it signals the brain that it is time to eat, sharpening appetite and increasing the secretion of gastric acid. It also stimulates peristalsis, the rippling motion of muscles in the stomach and intestine. An easy way to remember the function of this peptide: "Ghrelin gets the stomach growlin.'"

Ghrelin levels play a role in determining how quickly hunger returns. Low ghrelin levels are also associated with insufficient sleep. This may help to explain why getting enough sleep is critical to resuming control over appetite. We'll explore how getting adequate sleep plays an important role in maintaining appetite control in Chapter 16.

High ghrelin levels challenge appetite control because they have a powerful effect on making high-calorie foods more appealing. The effects of high ghrelin levels mimic the effects of fasting, so urgent is the desire for food. In one study, a dose of ghrelin was administered to half of a group of healthy volunteers; the other group had placebo. High-calorie foods were more difficult to resist among those who had taken ghrelin. The researchers explained that the part of the brain known as the orbital frontal cortex, involved in encoding the reward value of food, was strongly stimulated by ghrelin. They concluded that ghrelin may underlie the biological basis of food's appeal, and that the degree to which we find foods pleasurable or irresistible may be determined by levels of ghrelin in our bodies.

The neuropeptide *leptin*, in contrast, turns off hunger. When researchers discovered this appetite-suppressing neuropeptide in 1994, they confirmed the hypothesis of a physiological basis for obesity. Leptin may help regulate ghrelin levels. When leptin levels are low, food seems more rewarding. With high leptin levels, the reward pathway signal is extinguished. High levels therefore decrease food intake, increase energy expenditure, and help lower body weight.

Low leptin levels, observed especially often in people who binge at night, increase hunger and stimulate the pleasure centers of the brain when food is present. Leptin can also challenge dieters. As fatty tissue is lost, leptin production diminishes, which leads to an even stronger urge for food.

The body's "adipostat," a sort of thermostat that monitors the level of fat in cells, is regulated by leptin. In general, the more body fat you have, the more leptin there is in your blood. However, many people who are overweight develop what is called *leptin resistance*; the brain does not pick up the signals that supposedly curb appetite.

This phenomenon also occurs in laboratory animals. One study showed that when laboratory rats were given leptin, they ate less, but this the effect lasted only two weeks, after which the leptin no longer signaled the rats' brains to stop eating. Leptin is not effective when taken as a supplement by people who have leptin resistance.

Neuropeptide Y (NPY), found in high concentrations in the hypothalamus, has just the opposite effect of leptin. While leptin signals the brain that you have eaten enough, NPY powerfully stimulates the desire to eat. In one study, when NPY was injected into the brains of rats that had just eaten their fill, it induced subsequent uncontrolled eating. Moreover, it increased the rats' cells' storage of fat and decreased the rate of fat burning. Other studies have shown that overweight rats have high NPY levels. NPY levels rise after food deprivation, prompting the animals to eat more to replenish fat stores. After repeated doses of NPY, the rats in these studies become overweight, demonstrating all of the expected hormonal and metabolic changes associated with obesity.

Peptide YY (PYY), in contrast, extinguishes hunger. It is secreted by the digestive tract in response to food to signal the brain that the stomach is full. PYY slows down gastric emptying and both pancreatic and gastric secretions, producing a sense of satiety. It also inhibits production of the hunger-promoting NPY. Injecting PYY into lab animals inhibits their intake of food and reverses weight gain. In the average person, PYY levels increase immediately after eating and remain elevated for as long as six hours. Low levels of PYY, on the other hand, take the brakes off appetite control and lead to disordered eating. In overweight people, levels of PYY are relatively low and in response to eating, less PYY is produced than in people of normal weight.

GABA, or gamma-aminobutyric acid, is the body's primary inhibitory neuropeptide. While excitatory peptides push a cell to action, inhibitory peptides calm you down. GABA is synthesized in the brain from glutamate with the aid of vitamin B6. It increases relaxation, reduces stress, and improves focus. GABA has been used to relieve anxiety, prevent convulsions, and elevate mood. Benzodiazepine medications such as Valium, Xanax, and Ativan work by stimulating the uptake of GABA.

Low GABA levels are present in people with diabetes and impaired glucose tolerance. These conditions force the body to secrete extra insulin to accomplish the task of getting rid of excess blood sugar. Afterward, if the kidneys and liver don't do away with the extra insulin quickly, the blood sugar will drop too low, increasing the appetite and the urge to binge. GABA can reduce an overactive appetite. Its calming effects can also help those who eat in response to stress, anxiety, or depression.

The neuropeptides, like the neurotransmitters, play a key role in appetite and appetite control. I briefly described a few peptides involved in appetite regulation, but there are actually many more. Our appetite is regulated by multiple complex neurochemical systems that have evolved to manage hunger. Although the science is complicated and a detailed analysis of the functions of many peptides is beyond the scope of this book, keep in mind that abnormal neuropeptide activity is a major factor in disordered eating. All neuropeptides are dependent on optimal availability of amino acids.

Tryptophan and 5-Hydroxytryptophan (5-HTP)

The amino acid *tryptophan* is the precursor from which serotonin is made. The body's synthesis of serotonin depends directly on the amount of tryptophan available in the brain. Serotonin has been called the master appetite controller, as it inhibits appetite by activating cells in the hypothalamus, an area of the brain responsible for satiety and calm. Merely the sight, smell, or thought of food causes a release of serotonin in the hypothalamus. As eating continues, serotonin levels continue to rise until you feel full and satisfied. Then, high levels of serotonin turn off the appetite. When the body does not get enough serotonin, binge eating, irritability, and anxiety can result. Serotonin deficiency is linked to the brain's perception of starvation and hunger.

Many research studies have confirmed a link between low tryptophan and poor appetite control. One study involving bulimic patients found that as tryptophan levels became depleted, meal size increased. After just one tryptophan-depleted meal, patients experienced a lower mood, were increasingly concerned about body image, and reported a loss of control over eating. In a study of overweight participants, tryptophan depletion significantly increased the participants' consumption of sweets, as well as the likelihood that they would choose to eat sweets before any other type of food. These studies show that supplying the brain with enough tryptophan, which is necessary for serotonin production, appears to be a key to appetite regulation, especially among those with a tendency to binge.

Tryptophan is found in large amounts in high-protein foods, most notably eggs, cheese, fish, poultry, beef, and soybeans. Once tryptophan enters the bloodstream it, like other amino acids, is sent wherever the body needs it most at the time: it may become part of a hormone, an enzyme, or another protein molecule. Then, when the body's other needs have been satisfied, most of the left-over tryptophan will be converted in the brain to *5-hydroxytryptophan* (5-HTP), which in turn will be converted to serotonin with the help of vitamin B6.

Conversion of amino acids into active neurotransmitters requires the availability of nutrient cofactors that are commonly depleted in individuals as a result of medications, dietary deficiencies, and environmental stress. By ensuring that vitamin and mineral cofactors are adequate, we can optimize neurotransmitter synthesis in the brain to help with reestablishing appetite control.

Vitamin B3, vitamin B6, vitamin B12 and L-methylfolate are important cofactors required to convert tryptophan into serotonin. Low levels of B3 will affect serotonin levels in two ways: first, the conversion of tryptophan to 5-HTP will be limited, since vitamin B3 facilitates this step. Secondly, the liver will take up even more tryptophan to compensate for the lack of the vitamin just to convert it to 5-HTP.

When vitamin B6 levels are low, the conversion of 5-HTP to serotonin will be disrupted and less than one percent of the amino acid will actually reach the brain. Low levels of vitamin B6 are usually observed in women who are pregnant, lactating, or taking oral contraceptives, or in individuals with alcohol and substance abuse dependencies. When vitamin B6 supplements were given to rats in a study, the amount of 5-HTP in these rats' brains was considerably higher than in those not receiving vitamin B6 supplementation.

L-methylfolate is a form of folate that readily crosses the blood-brain barrier for use in neurotransmitter production. L-methylfolate is able to increase folate concentrations in the central nervous system, and it plays an active role in the crucial steps of serotonin and dopamine synthesis. Individuals deficient in L-methylfolate cannot utilize tryptophan appropriately to synthesize serotonin.

Deficiencies in amino acids and vitamin and mineral cofactors may result in decreased production of critical chemicals that affect mood and appetite. Without sufficient cofactors to ensure optimal utilization of amino acids for neurotransmitter synthesis, disordered eating behavior may follow. Conversion of 5-HTP to serotonin will not occur in the absence of these vital cofactors.

For many years, clinicians have found that 5-HTP is effective in treating anxiety and depression. Newer studies have shown that 5-HTP may also help with appetite and weight loss. Research results as to the effects of 5-HTP on disordered eating are encouraging. The first and most compelling research into the connection between 5-HTP and weight loss has come from Italy. The original Italian study was carried out with twenty overweight women. Half took 5-HTP; the other half received a placebo. The subjects' diets were not restricted. At the end of the study, those taking

5-HTP had lost more weight than the control group and also had consumed significantly fewer calories from carbohydrates—that is, they were eating less starchy, sugary food and less food overall.

The same research team undertook a second study to determine whether 5-HTP would lead to the same positive results with caloric restrictions. The first part of the study was arranged identically to the original study. Then, during a second 6 weeks, a 1,200 calorie diet was recommended and carbohydrate-rich snacks were prohibited. Patients taking 5-HTP lost an average of four pounds during the first six weeks and nearly twelve pounds during the second six-week period. Patients on placebo lost an average of less than one pound during the duration of the study. Although it might at first seem unsurprising that a calorie-restricted and carbohydrate-free diet would lead to weight loss, the difference in results between the 5-HTP group, who lost sixteen pounds in three months and the control group, who lost just two pounds, is both striking and promising.

More recently, scientists from the University of Pavia in Italy tested the use of sublingual 5-HTP spray on twenty-seven healthy but overweight adult women. The study subjects used either the spray or a spray that contained placebo under the tongue five times a day. Researchers found that the women using the spray with 5-HTP felt a greater sense of fullness than the control group. The 5-HTP group also completed the study with a lower age body mass index than the placebo group.

All of the current research supports the theory that supplying the brain with sufficient 5-HTP can help increase serotonin levels and regulate the appetite. More research for binge eating is clearly needed; however, 5-HTP has been useful as an adjunct to treatment, particularly when it is combined with another essential amino acid, phenylalanine.

Phenylalanine

Another essential amino acid with an important role in appetite control is phenylalanine. *Phenylalanine* is the precursor for two important neurotransmitters: dopamine and norepinephrine. Norepinephrine is a neurotransmitter that prompts a constellation of reactions collectively labeled the stress response. In times of stress, your heart beats faster, your blood pressure rises, and you accelerate your rate of breathing to enhance mental alertness and trigger the release of glucose into your bloodstream for quick energy. If you experience chronic stress, a sufficient supply of phenylalanine is necessary. Symptoms of phenylalanine deficiency include increased appetite, poor energy, depression, lack of alertness, and memory problems.

Phenylalanine comes in two forms, D and L, which are mirror images in terms of molecular structure. The D form is manufactured in a laboratory; the L form is natural. It is the L form that is useful as an appetite suppressant.

Phenylalanine acts in three ways to control appetite. First, it is the precursor to the synthesis of dopamine. Dopamine improves mood and decreases the urge to binge. Secondly, phenylalanine helps stimulate the production of the hormone *cholecystokinin* (CCK). This is the hormone that closes the valve leading from your stomach to your small intestine, inducing a feeling of fullness. When CCK is released, the brain receives a signal that the stomach is full. The third benefit of phenylalanine for appetite control is related to stimulation of the thyroid hormones. Phenylalanine is the precursor to tyrosine, and tyrosine is the amino acid required to manufacture thyroxine, the thyroid hormone that is essential in regulating the metabolic rate of the body.

Research in animals fed a diet high in L-phenylalanine showed a significant increase in the release of CCK and a significant decrease in food intake. Later, in a study of six normal-weight, fasting men, half were given 10 grams of L-phenylalanine twenty minutes before a meal, while the other half took a placebo. Men taking the L-phenylalanine consumed approximately one-third fewer calories than men in the control group because they reported greater feelings of fullness. Finally, a study of L-phenylalanine's effect on food intake in women showed that taking L-phenylalanine reduced caloric intake at lunch and dinner by ten percent and total daily caloric intake by nine percent.

Phenylalanine inhibits the appetite and decreases food intake by inducing a feeling of fullness. It is important to note, however, that only the L form of phenylalanine induces the release of CCK and helps to depress the appetite. Phenylalanine supplements should always have the L form in the combination known as DL-phenylalanine.

Tyrosine

A third key amino acid related to appetite is *tyrosine*. This nonessential amino acid is derived from phenylalanine and easily passes into the brain through the blood-brain barrier. There it is converted to dopamine and the stress hormones norepinephrine and epinephrine. Tyrosine has various functions. Tyrosine is the precursor for thyroxine, the thyroid hormone that helps control metabolic rate, growth rate, and mental health. Tyrosine also helps ward off stress-related depression.

Because of tyrosine's wide-ranging effects on the body in general and on neurotransmitters in particular, low levels of this amino acid can lead to several problems. A lack of dopamine increases the risk of addictive behaviors such as bingeing, drug use, alcoholism, and risk taking. Too little norepinephrine can interfere with appetite control, increasing hunger while preventing the breakdown of fat stores. As the body's stress hormones become more and more depleted, the risk of depression increases, which can cause appetite disturbances ranging from no appetite at all to intense cravings and bingeing.

There are only a few studies on tyrosine's direct effect upon the appetite. Animals fed a meal high in tyrosine released higher amounts of CCK and ate less than the control group, although the results seen with tyrosine were not as significant as those seen with L-phenylalanine. Results of a study involving mice suggest that supplemental tyrosine may help ease the cognitive and mood problems associated with maintaining a newly reduced body weight after dieting. Researchers induced stress in the mice by separating them, which depleted their dopamine and norepinephrine levels, well-known causes of mood problems. However, when the mice were given supplemental tyrosine, their levels returned to normal.

The *Journal of Psychiatry and Neuroscience* reported that L-Tyrosine has been a topic of major interest for many military research studies for its ability to reduce stress. Many animal studies show that the level of L-Tyrosine in the brain influences the amount of dopamine and norepinephrine available, which affect mood and alertness. During physical stress, brain neurons are firing rapidly, and this depletion can be normalized by L-Tyrosine supplementation. Dr. Simon Young reports that military test subjects have continued to respond positively to L-Tyrosine supplementation under physical duress. One study investigated whether tyrosine would be able to counteract the adverse environmental conditions with which military personnel are commonly faced. Military personnel were given 1,000 milligrams of L-Tyrosine or a placebo and subsequently exposed to cold and hypoxia. The military personnel who received L-Tyrosine reported fewer adverse side effects and improved cognitive function and mood as compared with those in the control group. L-Tyrosine can be of important benefit to individuals struggling with the effects of environmental stress factors, such as an uncontrollable appetite. In Chapter 14, you will learn more on how stress can hinder digestion and absorption of nutrients, disrupting your body's ability to regulate eating behavior. Relaxation is key when trying to reestablish appetite control.

Glutamine

Glutamine is the most abundant amino acid in the body. Glutamine removes the body's common waste product, ammonia, aids in immune system function, promotes normal digestion, plays an important part in brain function, serves as a metabolic fuel, and acts as a precursor to other amino acids and to glucose. It is converted into the excitatory neurotransmitter *glutamate*, one of the most important neurotransmitters for regulating normal brain function.

Glutamine primarily affects appetite through its role as metabolic fuel for glucose. When the body experiences a shortfall in glucose, it sends powerful signals demanding pumped-up glucose levels. The usual response is to eat sugary foods. Taking glutamine can achieve the same effect. Glutamine suppresses the release of insulin, which halts the decline in blood sugar levels. It also stimulates the release of glycogen and promotes the formation of blood sugar in the liver and kidneys, both of which help refuel the brain. When a person deficient in glutamine takes supplements of this amino acid, sugar cravings diminish.

Glutamine supplies can easily be depleted by stress, whether the stress is due to injuries, burns, surgery, trauma, or exhaustive exercise. Stress provokes the release of the hormone cortisol, which depletes glutamine supplies and impairs immunity. Conversely, glutamine supplements strengthen the immune system and reduce infections. Endurance athletes in training typically have depleted glutamine supplies, which may explain why they often develop colds after an event.

Your brain is fueled by glucose and needs a constant supply of it. Any shortfall in fuel is considered an emergency by the brain, which sends powerful messages urging you to eat foods that can quickly increase blood glucose levels. The quickest way to increase glucose and fuel the brain is to eat sugary foods. Glutamine helps replenish glucose supplies to the brain, stabilizing mood and preventing sugar cravings and bingeing. If you have a problem with hypoglycemia or sugar/carbohydrate cravings, supplemental glutamine may help.

Glycine

A nonessential amino acid manufactured from the amino acids serine and threonine, *glycine* helps convert glucose into energy, maintain the digestive and central nervous systems, and create DNA and RNA, the genetic blueprints for every cell in the body. Glycine also helps form and sustain muscle tissue by increasing levels of the muscle-building compound creatine. Because glycine makes up nearly one-third of the body's collagen, it is instrumental in the repair of damaged tissue. It also helps relieve muscle spasticity when combined with the amino acid taurine. Glycine is a *glucogenic amino acid*, which means it can create glucose when the body needs it. It also aids in digestion by regulating the manufacture of bile acids, used to break down fats. By modulating certain neuropeptides, glycine can also help normalize sleep patterns and circadian rhythms. It has proved useful in easing the onset of sleep, stabilizing sleep states and reducing daytime fatigue. Glycine helps keep blood sugar stable by mobilizing *glycogen*, a stored carbohydrate released into the bloodstream as glucose. It recharges energy levels and helps ward off sugar cravings, bingeing, hypoglycemia, and chronic fatigue syndrome.

Taurine

Taurine is a nonessential amino acid manufactured from methionine and cysteine in the presence of vitamin B6. Taurine helps regulate the nervous system and plays an important role in modulating our stress response. Taurine is an inhibitory amino acid that balances the excitatory effects of norepinephrine and epinephrine. Taurine supports mental performance and has antioxidant properties, which is why it is commonly found in energy drinks. While taurine can be obtained by eating meat and fish, it is better known as a dietary supplement for athletes and those trying to improve concentration.

The few research studies of taurine and appetite have yielded intriguing results. A study of satiety involving twenty-five healthy subjects explored the effects of a normal soy protein breakfast compared to a high soy protein breakfast. The high soy protein breakfast produced higher postmeal concentrations of taurine and insulin and was rated as more filling than the normal soy protein breakfast. Researchers concluded that the greater satiety resulted from elevated taurine and insulin levels.

A 2006 study conducted in Japan found that taurine deficiency creates a vicious circle that promotes obesity. Taurine is broken down by an enzyme called *cysteine dioxygenase* (CDO), which is found in large amounts in white adipose tissue (belly fat). In overweight mice, high levels of CDO lowered blood levels of taurine. But when the mice were given supplemental taurine, their metabolism increased, and the obesity normally induced by a high-fat diet was prevented. The researchers concluded that too little taurine may promote obesity, which further depletes taurine through the production of CDO. Dietary taurine supplementation interrupts this vicious circle.

Taurine's possible effect as an anti-obesity agent at the cellular level has been studied. In one study, thirty college students with a body mass index over 25 kg/m were randomly assigned to take 3 grams of taurine or a placebo orally for seven weeks. At the end of the study, triacylglycerol levels and body weight were significantly reduced in the group who took taurine. These results suggest that taurine may have beneficial effects on lipid metabolism and thereby help overweight people lose weight. Taurine has a calming and stabilizing effect on the brain and may help increase the sense of satiety.

Arginine

L-arginine is an amino acid naturally produced by the body. It can also be obtained through foods such as dairy products, beef, and some seafood. L-arginine is a precursor to nitric acid production, which helps with dilation of the blood vessels.

The hypothesis that arginine supplementation may increase an individual's ability to burn fat by stimulating nitric oxide production was tested on genetically overweight animals called Zucker diabetic fatty rats. Half of the study rats were given drinking water containing arginine for ten weeks; the other group was given a placebo. At the end of the tenth week, the body weights of arginine-treated rats were sixteen percent lower than those of control rats. The results suggest that arginine supplementation may enhance nitric oxide synthesis to promote fat reduction.

Arginine supplementation may also improve insulin sensitivity in people who are not overweight but who have diabetes. Participants with both diabetes and insulin resistance were divided into two groups: the first was treated with arginine, while the second was given placebo. Both groups ate low-calorie diets and participated in an exercise program; people in both groups lost weight, but those whose diets were supplemented with L-arginine lost more body weight and had greater decreases in waist circumference than those who took placebo.

Currently, arginine is produced in supplement pills and powders and added to most pre-workout drinks in combination with other performance enhancers. As we age, our bodies' ability to synthesize arginine decreases. Many anti-aging clinics use arginine to help combat negative effects of aging, though few scientific studies have conclusively proven these effects.

Branched Chain Amino Acids

The amino acids leucine, isoleucine and valine are collectively known as *branched chain amino acids* (BCAAs). The term *branched chain* refers to their unique chemical structure, which includes a characteristic side chain that stems out into links of carbon atoms. Together, these three essential compounds make up about thirty-five percent of the amino acids found in muscle proteins, where they play a crucial role in protein synthesis and metabolism.

The branched chain amino acids are closely involved in the creation and breakdown of proteins in the body. By activating various enzymes, the BCAAs help to turn on and off your body's ability to create proteins. Maintaining adequate protein production is not only necessary for muscle building, but is also vital for proper growth and development, nervous system function, and recovery from illness or injury. Studies of the branched-chain amino acid L-leucine conclude that it reduces both food intake and body weight in rats.

In October 2013, findings published in *Diabetes, Metabolic Syndrome and Obesity: Targets and Therapy* demonstrated that supplementation with a combination of leucine and vitamin B6 resulted in significant weight loss ranging from fifty to eighty percent over a twenty-four-week period in overweight participants. Participants were given a nutraceutical containing 2.25 grams of leucine and 30 milligrams of vitamin B6 or a placebo. Those who took the supplement lost up to twice as much weight as those who took the placebo. The effectiveness of the supplement is driven mainly by leucine's ability to decrease fat storage and B6's ability to stimulate muscle fat oxidation.

Scientists from the University of California's Genome Research Institute demonstrated that the signaling pathway *mTOR*, which is activated by nutrient and hormonal signals, plays a role in alerting the brain as to how much energy the body has available. These findings suggest that *mTOR* serves as a checkpoint for picking up energy changes that could be manipulated to adjust food intake. This pathway is also sensitive to BCAA, particularly leucine. When leucine was administered directly to the hypothalamus in the rats' brains, scientists observed reduced food intake. Though the findings are preliminary, these results make a convincing case that diets should integrate micronutrients and amino acids, which may be responsible for driving certain pathways in the brain that regulate appetite and body weight.

By modulating protein synthesis, the BCAAs directly affect your body's responses to food intake and the regulation of appetite and weight. When nutrients become available, the BCAAs initiate two signaling systems, which stimulate the hypothalamic region in the brain to decrease appetite and simultaneously rev up protein metabolism.

Simultaneously, the BCAAs help to regulate glucose levels, even in the absence of insulin, by accelerating the use of glucose by the liver. Through a combination of these functions, the BCAAs help your body facilitate energy metabolism by keeping weight and appetite in check. Branched chain amino acids help regulate protein synthesis and metabolism while also decreasing appetite and stabilizing glucose levels. They help decrease cravings, regulate blood sugar, and ease the stress hormone response.

James Greenblatt, MD

Why Amino Acid Levels Are Too Low

If amino acids are basic nutritional elements produced within our bodies or ingested through the food we eat, why do so many people lack the necessary amino acids to help regulate appetite? Several factors can contribute to an amino acid deficiency. Perhaps the main general cause is that many people living in westernized cultures today simply don't consume enough protein. Vegans, vegetarians, and those adolescents who subsist on a diet of pasta are at greatest risk.

Another contributing factor is poor digestion of protein. This is discussed in more detail in Chapter 10. Protein is broken down in the stomach, which secretes *hydrochloric acid*. This powerful acid converts a substance called pepsinogen into pepsin, an enzyme that reduces protein into smaller components, called polypeptides. Without enough hydrochloric acid, protein digestion is inefficient. Hydrochloric acid also helps with the absorption of vitamin B12 and certain minerals and triggers the satiety signal. Too little hydrochloric acid prevents absorption of these nutrients and weakens the signal to the brain that the belly is full.

A third factor is age. As we age, stomach acid levels decrease. They drop by almost forty percent from the teens to the thirties and almost half again by the seventies. Consequently, our ability to digest protein diminishes with age.

Antacids can further deplete amino acid levels. Millions of people who experience stomach discomfort and develop indigestion from overeating treat themselves with antacids. Taking antacids actually makes the situation worse. People trying to medicate their discomfort may unwittingly exacerbate problems with protein digestion by reducing their already low levels of hydrochloric acid even further. As stomach acid in fact helps control appetite, decreasing levels can reinforce disordered patterns of eating.

Treatment with Amino Acids

Although eating a diet rich in protein is important, my first recommendation to those struggling with disordered eating is to try amino acid supplements. Hundreds of patients have reported that intense cravings for food subsided soon after they began taking amino acid supplements.

It is best to start with a free-form amino acid blend of all the essential amino acids. A free-form blend bypasses the digestion process and is easily absorbed by the body to be used in protein, neuropeptide, and neurotransmitter synthesis. The blend of all the essential amino acids provides a foundation on which you can build a targeted treatment program.

In addition, I recommend a combination of 5-HTP and DL-phenylalanine. This combination increases serotonin, dopamine, and CCK, providing a simple way to influence the complex pathways of neurotransmission and appetite. Often, these two amino acids along with the blend of free form amino acids will be sufficient to help you take back control over your appetite and get off the roller coaster.

Amino acids are easy to take, and laboratory tests are not needed before you begin. Supplements are available in both pill and powder form. A woman should take a maximum of 10 grams of amino acid blend three times a day; a man can take 15 grams three times a day. To make sure the supplements are fully absorbed, take them at least thirty minutes before any meal or two hours after.

Although lab tests are not necessary to perform before taking amino acids, personalized supplementation based on fasting amino acid testing is always preferable. It is always best to find a physician or other healthcare provider who is knowledgeable about potential side effects and drug interactions. If you are taking prescription antidepressant medications that contain monoamine oxidase (MAO) inhibitors, you should not use amino acid supplements.

Amino acid supplements are often the most important factor toward optimizing appetite control, decreasing bingeing and sugar cravings, improving mood, and diminishing anxiety. Time and again, I have watched patients enjoy success with getting their eating patterns under control after they have begun taking amino acids.

All aspects of physiological and biochemical appetite control involve amino acids. From a single amino acid to more complicated peptides, neurotransmitters, and hormones, amino acids serve as foundations for the vast majority of the biochemistry behind appetite control. By optimizing amino acid levels, you will be able to synthesize both simple and complicated proteins that are required to maintain hunger management and normalize eating behavior. The first steps to take immediately after optimizing digestion with digestive enzymes are:

1. Utilize free form amino acids that are easily absorbed by the body to provide all the essential amino acids, such as tryptophan, to serve as precursors for important neurotransmitter synthesis.
2. Try targeted amino acid supplementation that incorporates 5-hydroxytryptophan (5-HTP) and DL-phenylalanine. This combination of single amino acids provides the most dramatic regulation of appetite by optimizing the synthesis of serotonin and peptides involved in appetite control.
3. For sugar cravings, try taking glutamine or glycine supplements. Many patients have found significant relief from adding these amino acids into their treatment.

Using amino acids is not a new medical breakthrough. The solution is logical, commonsense, and easy. If a nutritional deficiency causes a problem, then supplementing the body with what it has been missing can solve it. Sometimes the most significant intervention for treatment of disordered eating is providing the body with adequate precursor amino acids. A major element of the New Hope model for restoring a healthy appetite is optimizing neurotransmitter and neuropeptide levels with amino acids. Sometimes the answer to binge eating is simple, and this is the only intervention needed.

New Hope Core Amino Acid Supplements

Supplement	Contains	Daily Dosage Instructions
Free-form essential amino acids	5-HTP, phenylalanine, tyrosine, glutamine, glycine, arginine, branched chain amino acids	10-15 grams/day (Approximately 2 teaspoons mixed with water or juice before meals)
Targeted amino acid precursors	5-HTP and dl-phenylalanine	5-HTP: 50-200 milligrams DL-phenylalanine: 300- 3,000 milligrams
Digestive enzymes with Betaine Hydrochloric Acid	Broad-spectrum plant-based digestive enzymes with Betaine Hydrochloric Acid	1-2 capsules with meals

Amino Acid Supplements for Sugar Cravings

Supplement	Contains	Daily Dosage Instructions
Glycine	Glycine	1-2 grams
Glutamine	Glutamine	500-1,000 milligrams three times a day

Amino Acid Supplements for Weight Management

Supplement	Contains	Daily Dosage Instructions
Taurine	Taurine	1-3 grams
Branched chain amino acids (BCAAs)	Leucine, isoleucine, valine	1-5 grams

Summary

Appetite is strongly influenced by three specific molecular structures in the body: peptides, hormones, and neurotransmitters. When these regulator molecules are in balance, hunger cues are natural and appropriate, eating patterns are synchronized, and appetite is generally under control. However, the body requires adequate amounts of raw material in the form of small organic compounds called amino acids to create these larger molecules at a steady rate. When there are insufficient amino acids present to meet demands, the production of peptides, hormones, and neurotransmitters falters, and appetite can quickly spiral out of control.

There are approximately twenty different types of amino acids that combine to create all of the functional proteins in the body. Some amino acids are manufactured by the body, while others, deemed essential amino acids, must be consumed through the diet. Each influences appetite and metabolism in a specific way—primarily through the modulation of neurotransmitter and hormone function. Tryptophan, for example, is the precursor to serotonin, while tyrosine helps to prevent stress-related depression by influencing dopamine, norepinephrine, and epinephrine levels. Glutamate is involved in the production of GABA, one of the body's primary calming neurotransmitters. Other amino acids impact appetite via their roles in glucose metabolism such as: carnitine, which helps glucose reach the cells; glycine, which mobilizes stored glucose for energy; and glutamine, which replenishes glucose supplies to the brain. The branched chain amino acids work to regulate protein synthesis and metabolism, thus also decreasing appetite and stabilizing glucose levels.

When taken properly, amino acids can help to recalibrate the underlying biochemical imbalances that distort appetite and exacerbate destructive eating patterns. Working with a qualified healthcare practitioner to replenish amino acid levels can be an empowering step in regaining appetite control.

Integrative Medicine for Binge Eating

Key Points

- Low levels of the neurotransmitters serotonin, dopamine, and norepinephrine can cause appetite disturbances and eating problems.
- All peptides, hormones, and neurotransmitters are manufactured from amino acids, the organic compounds that combine to create proteins.
- There are approximately twenty different amino acids, distinguished between "essential" amino acids and "nonessential" amino acids. Our body is capable of making essential amino acids on its own, while the nonessential amino acids must be obtained through diet.
- When amino acids are in short supply, neurotransmitter production decreases and hormone levels become imbalanced.
- Amino acid supplements provide the raw material needed to increase the production of neurotransmitters, peptides, and hormones, which may calm appetite problems.
- Supplying the brain with sufficient tryptophan (in the form of 5-HTP) can help increase serotonin levels and regulate appetite, especially among those with a tendency to binge.
- Phenylalanine inhibits appetite and decreases food intake by inducing a feeling of fullness.
- Tyrosine helps ward off stress-related depression as well as bingeing that is related to too little dopamine, norepinephrine, or epinephrine.
- GABA, known for its calming and relaxing effects, is helpful for those who eat in response to stress, anxiety, or depression. It also lowers the body's need for insulin, helping to prevent blood sugar crashes that can lead to bingeing behavior.
- Glutamine helps replenish glucose supplies to the brain, stabilizing the mood and preventing sugar cravings and bingeing.
- Glycine helps keep blood sugar stable by mobilizing glycogen, a stored carbohydrate that is released into the bloodstream as glucose. Glycine helps improve energy and ward off sugar cravings, bingeing, and hypoglycemia.

- Taurine provides a calm and stabilizing effect on the brain to help increase satiety.
- Branched chain amino acids help regulate protein synthesis and metabolism, while also decreasing appetite and stabilizing glucose levels.

10
CONTROLLING APPETITE WITH VITAMIN AND MINERAL SUPPLEMENTS

A metabolic assessment is rarely integrated into a psychiatric evaluation. Many mental health professionals and psychiatrists are just beginning to understand how important nutrition may be for optimal brain functioning and mental health. Rather than treating symptoms alone, the most effective treatment targets nutritional and metabolic imbalances that are interfering with your body's ability to regulate appetite. Once balance is restored, the symptoms often diminish or even disappear.

In Chapter 8, I discussed tests that can help you discover underlying nutritional deficiencies that may be contributing to your health and appetite disturbances. Some of these problems, such as thyroid abnormalities, will require medical attention. But others are responsive to nutritional supplements. I suggest that you work with a healthcare provider familiar with biochemical individuality to create an individualized supplement program based on the results of your metabolic tests. Don't try to figure it out yourself, as overloading on supplements or taking supplements you don't need can be both expensive and frustrating, and lead to another journey toward failure.

A comprehensive metabolic evaluation is a critical part of restoring appetite control. After you have repleted all nutritional deficiencies, the addition of core New Hope supplements will support neurotransmitter synthesis and minimize the out-of-control appetite that prompts disordered eating. Over many years of clinical experience, I have found these nutritional supplements invaluable in the treatment of eating disorders. When your body is provided with the right nutrients, you are better equipped to achieve success and regain control over your appetite, cravings and binge eating.

In addition to the amino acids discussed in Chapter 9, the core nutritional program for the New Hope model incorporates the following nutrients:

- Digestive enzymes
- Probiotics
- B vitamins
- L-methylfolate
- Trace minerals (zinc, chromium, magnesium)
- Essential fatty acids
- Curcumin
- Inositol

A targeted nutritional supplement for sugar cravings is:

- Gymnema

Digestive Enzymes

Recovery from disordered eating depends on a healthy digestive system. I often see patients who eat healthy diets consisting of organic foods and adequate protein, whose blood work nevertheless reveals that they are, in fact, malnourished. Nutritional status is not based on *what* you eat. Instead, it depends upon your *ability to digest and absorb* nutrients from food.

A healthy digestive system is like a well-oiled machine with smooth transitions between its several phases of operation. When you see a plate of food, smell its aroma, and think about the first bite, chemical messengers in the brain send signals to the digestive system. After food is swallowed, it travels down the esophagus and into the stomach, helped along by rhythmic contractions of the ring-like muscles in the esophagus. Once the food arrives in the stomach, the stomach's expansion triggers secretion of digestive enzymes and gastric acid. The stomach chemically and mechanically transforms the food into a liquid mixture, composed of partially digested food, water, digestive enzymes, and *hydrochloric acid* (HCL). The extremely acidic nature of HCL is essential for proper digestion, as it helps break down protein, absorb vitamins and minerals, and communicate to the brain that you are full. In other words, hydrochloric acid is good for digestion.

If you have digestive troubles, especially *gastroesophageal reflux disease* (GERD), you may have developed the habit of taking antacids. And if so, you're not alone. Each year, more than sixty million prescriptions are written for medications designed to lower or neutralize stomach acid, and that number doesn't include the mountain of over-the-counter antacids routinely purchased and used indiscriminately.

The widespread popularity of antacids is based on the fallacy that hydrochloric acid is a "bad" thing. Many people don't realize that HCL, in addition to its other essential functions, communicates satiety to the brain. The symptoms of low stomach acid are, ironically, much like the problems that people try to remedy by taking antacids: bloating, flatulence, food sensitivities, and pain or discomfort after eating. Low stomach acid prevents nutrients from being absorbed, and poor nutrient status can render the stomach incapable of producing enough acid. Add antacids to the mix, and the problem spirals.

After digestion in the stomach is finished, the liquid mixture is pushed slowly to the small intestine. This is where most of the digestion of proteins, fats, and carbohydrates occurs. Partially-digested protein is broken into single amino acids. Bile released from the gallbladder breaks fat into smaller droplets, and pancreatic enzymes break those droplets into monoglycerides and fatty acids. Simplified forms of protein, fat, and carbohydrates are absorbed through the walls of the small intestine and then transported into the bloodstream. Most vitamins and minerals are also absorbed in the small intestine. Therefore, the health of the small intestine is a critical determining factor in nutrient absorption.

The body's production of digestive enzymes depends upon the presence of enough nutrients, including vitamins, zinc, and amino acids. Poor nutrition causes inefficient digestion, which leads to poor absorption of the nutrients digested, resulting in even less efficient digestion. While I suggest that you minimize antacid use, you should supplement your diet with digestive enzymes to maximize digestion and nutrient absorption.

The supplemental digestive enzyme combination should be a broad-spectrum type that helps you digest carbohydrates, proteins, and fat. The number of enzymes each individual should take varies according to diet, lifestyle, and biochemical individuality. For people with binge eating disorder, the digestive enzyme combination should include Betaine HCL, essential for breaking protein down into precursor amino acids that are required for the synthesis of appetite-regulating neurotransmitters and peptides.

If you have an ulcer, do not take HCL. If you experience a burning sensation in your stomach, do not continue HCL supplements.

DPP-IV Enzyme (Dipeptidyl Peptidase)

As discussed in Chapter 8, the body requires a special digestive enzyme called *dipeptidyl peptidase* (DPP-IV) that is used to break down casein and gluten peptides into individual amino acids for the body to use. Some individuals are DPP-IV deficient, and others may consume so much casein- and gluten-containing food that demand exceeds the supply of available DPP-IV enzyme. DPP-IV supplementation can assist in the proper digestion of dairy and gluten products.

DPP-IV requires adequate amounts of zinc in order to function properly. Vegans and vegetarians are at a higher risk of having zinc deficiencies, as they avoid meat products which are the main dietary sources of zinc. It is important to make sure that you are tested for zinc deficiency if you are experiencing issues with digestion.

Without DPP-IV enzyme to break down casein and gluten, the build-up of casomorphin and gliadorphin can cause food cravings and mood disturbances. For many of you, taking one to two capsules of DPP-IV enzyme with meals can provide tremendous benefit.

Probiotics

Your appetite depends in part upon the proper functioning of your intestines, and one of the key ways to improve intestinal function is through the use of probiotics. *Probiotics* are "good" bacteria that help the body digest and absorb vitamins, fatty acids, and other nutrients. The human intestinal tract is home to as many as one hundred trillion microorganisms, which may include bacteria, fungi, archaea, and protozoans and which, together, are known as the *gut microbiota*. The quality, quantity, and physiologic activity of the microbiota can easily be changed for the worse by antibiotics, birth control pills, laxative abuse, poor nutrition, and stress. As levels of symbiotic microbes – particularly bacteria, which dominate the gut microbiota - fluctuate, there can be a corresponding increase in physical and psychological problems, including changes in appetite and weight.

Probiotics provide many health benefits. In addition to promoting healthy digestion, they can reduce symptoms of colitis, irritable bowel syndrome, and yeast infections. Recent research has shown that probiotics and probiotic supplements can also help curb sugar cravings, resulting in stable blood sugar levels and weight loss. Although scientists are still uncertain as to the exact mechanism by which this occurs, they speculate that the probiotics feed on carbohydrates. As these friendly bacteria feed on sugars, they essentially use up the excess supply, thereby stabilizing blood sugar and minimizing the highs and lows that trigger mood swings, energy loss, and weight gain. This research suggests that probiotic supplementation, in tandem with eating probiotic-rich foods, can facilitate weight loss.

Studies with overweight patients have shown probiotic supplementation can produce a significant decrease in sugar cravings in as few as four days. Probiotics contain plentiful amounts of bacteria that can "seed" the intestines and promote the multiplication of these helpful organisms. Probiotic-containing foods include fermented foods such as yogurt and kefir, sauerkraut, kimchi, tempeh, miso, and kombucha. Probiotic supplements, however, offer much more concentrated doses of bacteria - sometimes numbering in the billions - and are therefore much more effective than probiotic-containing foods at restoring the intestinal microbiota. Probiotics are especially beneficial when appetite disturbances are related to digestive problems. But they can also help ease eating disturbances in two surprising ways: by enhancing mood and by making metabolism more efficient.

Recent research has shown that probiotics can have a favorable effect on mood. In animals, probiotics such as *Bifidobacteria infantis* suppress the inflammatory response and, at the same time, increase tryptophan levels. In humans, a study involving 124 healthy people found that consumption of a milk drink containing probiotics improved mood in those whose mood was initially poor. And in a 2009 study that followed thirty-nine chronic fatigue patients for two months, those who were given a daily probiotic (*Lactobacillus casei*) experienced a significant decrease in anxiety symptoms.

About ninety percent of intestinal bacteria belong to one of two groups: *Firmicutes* or *Bacteroidetes*. Those in the *Firmicutes* group are particularly good at extracting energy from food, which means they are very efficient at converting food into calories, a characteristic that may contribute to weight gain. At the same time, *low* levels of certain members of the *Bacteroidetes* group will increase the likelihood of leaky gut syndrome and inflammation, two conditions associated with weight and appetite disturbances. Scientific evidence suggests that the quality and quantity of microorganisms in the gut in both humans and animals are different in the lean than in the overweight, citing a relationship between bacteria and disordered eating behavior. Research has shown that overweight individuals have much greater amounts of *Firmicutes* and lesser amounts of *Bacteroidetes* than their lean counterparts. But when these overweight individuals lose weight, the proportions of bacteria shift and begin to resemble those of lean people.

Knowing that overweight people have more *Firmicutes* and fewer *Bacteroidetes* raises the question: if you change the proportions of their microflora to resemble those seen in their lean counterparts, will the overweight lose weight? In animal studies, researchers did just that. Overweight mice were given their regular chow mixed with bacteria from the *Bacteroidetes* family for a period of eight weeks. The mice lost weight and fatty tissue, even though their caloric intake was not decreased. In another study, researchers transferred the *Firmicutes*-rich intestinal bacteria from overweight mice into lean mice. The lean mice became overweight without increasing their calorie intake.

Studies that involve shifting types of bacteria in humans have shown encouraging results. Researchers experimented with a naturally occurring sugar called *oligofructose* that is known to increase levels of *Bifidobacteria*, a member of the *Bacteroidetes* group. In a study of normal-weight people, a two-week treatment with oligofructose increased satiety after breakfast and dinner, markedly reduced hunger and food consumption after dinner, and lowered total daily energy intake by approximately five percent. In a longer study, this one involving overweight adults, a twelve-week trial of supplementation with oligofructose promoted weight loss, improved glucose regulation, suppressed ghrelin, and enhanced *Peptide PYY* (PYY). PYY is a peptide that reduces appetite and plays an important role in increasing digestion and nutrient absorption after a meal by slowing the gastric emptying.

More research is being conducted to explore the effects of probiotics on obesity, but initial studies have yielded promising results. This approach to weight loss and hunger management is beneficial with probiotic supplementation of 50-100 billion CFUs per day.

B Vitamins

The B vitamins are important for normalizing eating patterns, as they help stabilize blood glucose levels. The vitamins that make up the B complex include thiamin, riboflavin, niacin, B6, B12, pantothenic acid, inositol, biotin, folic acid, and others that work together to convert carbohydrates into glucose, which means they help provide energy, decrease sugar cravings, fight fatigue, and ease hypoglycemia-related mood swings. These vitamins are also important in preventing depression. For example, at least four different double-blind studies have found that boosting thiamin levels lifts the mood of study participants. Additionally, vitamin B6 supplementation has been shown to stabilize mood in depressed patients; folic acid supplements given to depressed patients shortened the patients' recovery time; and mood and memory has improved in patients given B12 supplements.

The B vitamins most important to the regulation of appetite include vitamin B6, vitamin B12, inositol, and folate. They can be taken as single supplements or, in many cases, taken together in the form of a B complex.

Vitamin B6 is involved in a wide variety of functions in the body. Like the other B vitamins, B6 aids in the extraction of energy from proteins, fats, and carbohydrates. It also plays a part in the manufacture of amino acids from carbohydrates, the conversion of glucose into a form used by the muscles, normal functioning of the nervous system, the production of red blood cells and antibodies, and the synthesis of more than sixty different hormones, neurotransmitters, enzymes, and prostaglandins.

Vitamin B6 is directly involved in the regulation of appetite, mood, and sleep through its role in the production of neurotransmitters, especially serotonin. Vitamin B6 is required as a co-factor for the conversion of 5-HTP to serotonin. Low levels of B6 are commonly observed in patients struggling with disordered eating patterns.

If laboratory testing reveals a B6 deficiency, my preference is to use *Pyridoxal-5'-phosphate* (P5P), the activated form of this B vitamin. Some people may have difficulty converting vitamin B6 into P5P to be used by the body. P5P is required for proper absorption of B12, magnesium, and gastric HCL. It is also an important coenzyme in the metabolism of carbohydrates, fats, and proteins.

My recommendation for vitamin B6 repletion is 50 milligrams of vitamin B6 twice a day as part of a B complex or multivitamin. However, if laboratory testing reveals that vitamin B6 levels are low, it is best to use the activated form of the vitamin, P5P, instead.

Taking more than 200 milligrams of B6 daily is not recommended, as it can cause numbness and tingling in the limbs.

Folate (L-methylfolate)

The B vitamin *folate*, also referred to as folic acid, is crucial to the growth and maintenance of all cells as well as the synthesis of DNA. It markedly affects the production of all new proteins, especially proteins with a fast turnover rate such as those found in red blood cells, the cells lining the digestive tract, and the cells of a growing fetus. Low folate levels can cause anemia, gastrointestinal upset, and major defects in the fetal brain and spine known as neural tube defects. Folate-deficient individuals can also develop elevated blood levels of homocysteine, a risk factor for cardiovascular disease and Alzheimer's disease.

Folate assists in the manufacture of serotonin, dopamine, and norepinephrine, and deficiencies are common in people with depression. Research has shown folate and depression severity to be inversely correlated; in other words, lower folate levels are associated with more severe depression. Numerous studies have also found that depressed people who have low folate levels respond more poorly to antidepressant treatment and relapse more frequently than others. Higher folate levels, on the other hand, are linked to lower depression risk and severity. Taking folate supplements seems to also enhance the effects of antidepressants and relieve depression more effectively than simply taking antidepressants alone. However, those with a specific biochemical makeup may respond best to a form of the vitamin called *L-methylfolate*.

Folate must be converted into L-methylfolate in order to cross the blood-brain barrier and be made available for neurotransmitter synthesis. Unfortunately, some people have genetic mutations called *methlentetrahydrofolate reductase* (MTHFR) *polymorphisms* that slow this conversion, putting them at a higher risk of developing depression and being chronically depressed than those who don't have this mutation.

Recent research has elucidated the relationship between body-mass index (BMI), MTFHR polymorphisms, and the efficacy of L-methylfolate. In 2012, George Papakostas, MD, presented his findings at the 164th Annual Meeting of the American Psychiatric Association citing that metabolic biomarkers such as inflammation, BMI, and MTHFR gene defects can predict L-methylfolate efficacy.

In the study, patients with SSRI-resistant major depressive disorder were randomized to receive one of three treatments during a sixty-day trial: (1) L-methylfolate 15 milligrams in addition to an antidepressant for sixty days; (2) placebo and an antidepressant for thirty days, followed by 30 milligrams of Deplin for the remaining thirty days; (3) placebo in addition to an antidepressant for sixty days. Obese patients who received the 15 milligrams of L-methylfolate along with an antidepressant reported significantly greater symptomatic improvements as compared to those who received placebo. As obesity is known to increase the risk of major depressive disorder and cause poor response to antidepressant treatment alone, these results show that individuals with a MTHFR genetic variant or with a BMI greater than 30 can benefit the most from L-methylfolate supplementation.

Besides MTHFR polymorphisms, folate deficiency can be caused by poor diet, B12 deficiency, antacids, oral contraceptives, antibiotics, anticonvulsants, and the use of alcohol or tobacco products.

Depending on an individual's symptoms and laboratory testing results, I recommend between 1 and 15 milligrams per day of L-methylfolate.

Trace Minerals

Numerous trace minerals are essential for human health and optimal brain function, and three of these are particularly helpful for the treatment of eating disturbances: *chromium*, which helps to regulate glucose and control the symptoms of depression; *magnesium*, which fights insulin-resistant hunger, depression, and anxiety; and *zinc*, which can be critical to the treatment of depression and the restoration of a normal appetite.

Zinc

The mineral zinc plays important roles in growth and development, neurologic function, the immune response, reproduction, and neurotransmitter synthesis. Vital chemical reactions involving nearly one hundred different enzymes, including digestive enzymes, cannot be catalyzed without zinc. Zinc is also critical to our senses of taste and smell, bone growth, the production of proteins, DNA synthesis, cell division, and wound healing.

Because the body cannot store zinc, daily intake is necessary. Symptoms of zinc deficiency include hair loss, skin lesions, acne, diarrhea, and depression. White marks on the fingernails are an early sign of zinc deficiency.

Low zinc status is also related to depression. Research has shown that people with major depression have zinc levels that are twelve to sixteen percent lower than those who are not depressed. A meta-analysis of seventeen studies including 1,643 depressed and 804 control participants concluded that participants with depression had lower serum zinc concentrations than controls. Many important enzymes responsible for regulating neurotransmitter function and appetite are zinc-dependent. Zinc deficiencies set off a cascade of other biological actions that impair the ability to control food intake.

Zinc can also augment the efficacy of antidepressants. Antidepressants have been shown to have limited utility. *Polypharmacy* – an increasingly common tactic that involves prescribing more medication to offset the side effects or bolster the efficacy of existing prescriptions - can lead to unpleasant side-effects, often with no corresponding increase in effectiveness. When depressed patients in one study were given 25 milligrams of supplemental zinc per day in addition to their antidepressant, their depressive symptoms diminished more than those who received a placebo with their antidepressant. Many studies have also highlighted zinc's ability to make antidepressants more effective for people who were previously nonresponsive to pharmaceutical treatments.

Depending on assessment of zinc status, I recommend 30-60 milligrams of zinc per day. Do not take more than 100 milligrams of zinc per day as side effects may occur, including dizziness, lethargy, nausea and vomiting. In addition, large doses of zinc can damage the liver and pancreas and interfere with absorption of iron and copper.

Chromium

Inadequate chromium levels result in carbohydrate cravings, impaired glucose tolerance, hypoglycemia, and depression. Chromium is an essential part of *glucose tolerance factor* (GTF), a compound that helps insulin move blood sugar into the cells. Chromium works with the insulin receptors on the cells, helping "open the doors" so that glucose can enter. And even though the body contains a very small amount of chromium, when its stores become depleted, the effectiveness of insulin and the body's ability to handle glucose can markedly decrease. Poorly controlled glucose levels, in turn, can result in sugar or carbohydrate cravings and an increase in hunger.

It's estimated that twenty-five to fifty percent of Americans are chromium-deficient due to low levels of this mineral in our soil and in the refined foods (e.g., sugar, white flour) that make up a large percentage of our diet. To make matters worse, the body becomes less efficient at absorbing chromium with age, and high-sugar diets can deplete chromium stores as the mineral is needed to metabolize sugar.

Chromium's ability to help insulin "feed cells" can decrease cravings, overeating, and bingeing. It may also help treat a form of depression called *atypical depression*, which is characterized by mood reactivity, increased appetite, carbohydrate cravings, and weight gain. In one study, overweight women with carbohydrate cravings were randomized to receive either 1,000 micrograms of chromium picolinate per day or a placebo for eight weeks. Compared to those who had taken placebo, the women who took supplemental chromium experienced significantly reduced hunger levels, food intake, and fat cravings, and displayed greater reductions in body weight.

In another eight-week study, patients with atypical depression who received 600 micrograms/day of chromium picolinate experienced a marked decrease in depressive symptoms compared to those receiving a placebo. Of eight patients who comprised a subgroup of overeaters, four experienced a complete disappearance of overeating by the end of the study, compared to just one of five in the placebo group. Chromium treatment has been shown to improve mood, appetite, and glucose regulation in various psychiatric and medical patient populations. The authors of this study propose that chromium may be useful in the treatment of binge eating disorder (BED).

In July 2013, findings from a pilot trial for binge eating disorder were published that supported the use of chromium for regulating appetite and promoting weight loss. In this six-month trial, twenty-four overweight adults with BED were randomly assigned to receive 1,000 micrograms of chromium/day, 600 micrograms of chromium/day, or a placebo. Lower glucose levels, reduced binge frequency, modest weight loss, and decreased symptoms of depression were observed in participants who received supplemental chromium.

Dosages used for repletion range from 200-500 micrograms of *chromium picolinate* (the most readily-absorbed form of supplemental chromium) two times a day.

Magnesium

Magnesium plays a vital role in many of the body's metabolic processes, including the conversion of protein, fat, and carbohydrates into energy. Moreover, magnesium is critical for the proper functioning of over three hundred enzymes, including those necessary for the synthesis of neurotransmitters such as serotonin. Common symptoms associated with magnesium deficiency include headaches, constipation, insomnia, premenstrual syndrome (PMS), fatigue, anxiety, insulin resistance, and sugar cravings.

Magnesium status is generally poor in the United States, with more than two-thirds of Americans failing to meet the RDA for magnesium and one-fifth getting less than half the recommended amount. It is one of the first minerals to be depleted when the body is under stress and one of the first eliminated from food during processing. People who consume a typical western diet – in other words, a diet high in fat, sugar, and refined grains – are likely not getting enough magnesium.

Poor magnesium intake is common in individuals who adhere to restrictive diets or consume diets high in refined carbohydrates. Magnesium deficiency can contribute to insulin resistance, which leads to a "gnawing" hunger. Magnesium supplements may be able to combat this condition. A study of sixty-three diabetic patients with low blood levels of magnesium showed that magnesium supplementation improved both insulin sensitivity and metabolic control.

Magnesium deficiency can also cause psychological conditions including depression, irritability, and anxiety. Research studies have shown that oral magnesium treatment can be particularly effective in treating major depression. For example, in a twelve-week study of patients who had diabetes, low magnesium levels, and newly diagnosed depression, magnesium supplements were found to be just as effective as the antidepressant imipramine in treating depressive symptoms.

Many forms of magnesium are available at health foods stores. I recommend using *magnesium glycinate* or *magnesium citrate*. Depending on the individual's degree of deficiency, I recommend 400-600 milligrams of supplemental magnesium per day. Magnesium oxide should be avoided since it is commonly used as an antacid to relieve heartburn or acid indigestion and is poorly absorbed.

Essential Fatty Acids

Necessary for several biological processes, the *essential fatty acids* (EFAs) can't be manufactured by the body, so they must be obtained through diet. There are two families of EFAs: the *omega-3s*, which are found primarily in fish or fish oil and can be created in the body from flax oil; and the *omega-6s*, which are found primarily in vegetable oils and grains.

Growth and development, brain and nerve function, the control of inflammation, and the regulation of metabolism all depend on sufficient amounts of omega-3s being present for use within the body. Low plasma levels of the omega-3 known as DHA are linked to low serotonin levels and an increase in suicide attempts. In adolescents, low levels of another omega-3, EFA, have also been correlated with depression, while higher levels of this fatty acid seem to protect against it. Several studies have found that taking EFA supplements can reduce depressive and aggressive symptoms as well as suicidal thinking.

Omega-6 fatty acids also play important roles in brain function, and they are necessary for normal growth and development, bone health, and metabolic regulation. However, omega-6 intake has risen steadily over the past century due to the increasing prevalence and usage of plant oils – including corn, cottonseed, safflower, and sunflower oils – in the western diet. High concentrations of omega-6s 'crowd out' omega-3s, which means that more and more people worldwide are now consuming diets that provide too many omega-6s and too few omega-3s.

An EFA deficiency or a skewing of the omega-6 : omega-3 ratio can contribute to depression, obesity, and blood sugar abnormalities, all of which can affect eating habits and appetite. People who follow restrictive diets or who simply cut back drastically on fat intake may find themselves deficient in EFAs. EFA deficiencies contribute to a slowed metabolism that often results in more rapid weight gain after periods of restriction. Those who consume a standard high fat, highly processed western diet are very likely to experience an imbalance in the optimal ratio of omega-3 to omega-6 fatty acids.

Numerous studies have shown that omega-3 supplements can be helpful in treating depression. As for the effects of omega-3s on eating disorders, a study of seven young patients with anorexia found that when the patients were given 1 gram of EPA per day, three recovered from the eating disorder and four improved.

Daily doses of a combination of 3 grams of omega-3s from fish oil and 1 gram of omega-6s from evening primrose oil or borage oil be helpful for individuals who are EFA deficient. It is also important to take adequate amounts of antioxidants along with EFAs: at least 500 milligrams of vitamin C and 400 IU vitamin E per day.

Curcumin

Recent studies reveal the healing powers of *curcumin*, a component of the common household spice turmeric. With antioxidant and anti-inflammatory properties, curcumin imitates the antidepressant actions of the prescription drugs fluoxetine and imipramine – without any of the side effects. It has also been touted as an anti-obesity agent for its ability to reduce body fat and inhibit weight gain. A study published in the *Journal of Nutrition* reported that mice fed a high-fat diet along with supplemental curcumin had decreased weight gain and lowered cholesterol levels. While more research is needed to validate the importance of dietary curcumin in helping to regain appetite control, extensive research has focused on curcumin's ability to combat symptoms of depression, a condition that often coexists with disordered eating.

Curcumin has been shown to improve depressed mood, sleep disturbances, and fatigue. People with depression tend to have increased inflammation and decreased neurogenesis, both of which can be restored to healthy levels by curcumin.

Curcumin can also boost levels of vital neurotransmitters in the central nervous system. The decreased pleasure and reward, as well as the feelings of stress, that accompany a major depressive episode can be traced to reduced levels of serotonin, dopamine, and noradrenaline. Curcumin increases levels of both serotonin and dopamine, and marginally increases levels of noradrenaline within the brain.

Animal studies reinforce findings of the effects of curcumin on depression. When rats were placed in stressful situations, those treated with curcumin displayed heightened motivation to escape. Curcumin also appears to protect against mitochondrial damage, a finding that is significant for depressed patients, who often display mitochondrial impairments.

Research supports the use of supplemental curcumin for a wide range of metabolic symptoms associated with depression. I recommend a minimum of 250 milligrams of curcumin daily to support appetite control.

Inositol

Inositol, also known as vitamin B8, is responsible for forming healthy cell membranes and maintaining nutrient transfer between cells. Inositol is converted into a substance that regulates the action of serotonin. Restoring normal levels of this vitamin may thus help alleviate psychiatric symptoms, including depression, feelings of panic, and obsessive thoughts.

Several studies demonstrate the effectiveness of inositol for depression. While some studies involved patients taking inositol as an adjunct to antidepressant medications, others compared the efficacy of inositol as a sole treatment versus a placebo. Both approaches yielded similar results: depression improved significantly when inositol was taken.

One study examined inositol's potency as a treatment for binge eating disorder. Twelve patients with bulimia and binge eating were given 18 grams of either inositol or placebo and monitored for six weeks. The group taking the inositol reported significant improvements in symptoms compared to the placebo group at the end of the trial, demonstrating that inositol can be useful in the treatment of disorders characterized by appetite dysregulation as well depression and obsessive-control disorder.

Present in the tissues of the brain, nerves, muscles, bones, heart, and reproductive system, inositol is a precursor to several "signaling" molecules that tell cells how to behave. Some molecular signaling involves the activation of serotonin receptors, which may help improve appetite balance and ease depression. Inositol can be synthesized by the body and by the bacteria in the intestinal tract.

Inositol enhances insulin sensitivity, which can produce more energy, reduce cravings, and suppress the desire to binge. It also participates in the action of serotonin. Inositol has been effective in treating many of the same psychiatric disorders that are linked to eating disorders and responsive to

SSRIs, including depression, anxiety, and obsessive-compulsive disorder. More than thirty years ago, scientists discovered that depressed people often have below-normal levels of inositol in their spinal fluid. Treating them with 6-12 grams of inositol per day raised these levels significantly and eased depression; when treatment was halted, however, the depression returned. In another study, when patients with OCD were given daily doses of 18 grams of inositol, they experienced significant improvement in symptoms.

I recommend one-half teaspoon (1.4 grams) of inositol in powder form, taken three times daily to start. The dosage can be slowly increased over two to four weeks to 8-12 grams per day. If the dosage is increased too quickly, gastrointestinal problems may occur. For sugar cravings, I recommend 1 teaspoon of inositol powder to be taken daily.

Gymnema

Gymnema sylvestre is a traditional Ayurvedic herb that is native to central and western India, Africa and Australia. Its Hindi name, "gurmar," means "destroyer of sugar." Commonly found in most health food stores the form of tea, it is considered to have antidiabetic properties and is used to control obesity. When the leaves are chewed, it interferes with the ability to taste sweetness. Gymnema can be helpful for suppressing sugar cravings.

The active property of gymnema is *gymnemic acid*, which delays glucose absorption in the blood. Because the molecular structure of gymnemic acid is similar to glucose, it can help curb sugar cravings by filling in the receptor locations of sweet taste buds. Though more research is needed, gymnema may be an alternative medicine to treat sugar cravings due to its efficacy in blocking sugar binding sites, and by preventing sugar molecules from accumulating in the body.

Gymnema tea is often found on the shelves of health food stores and is promoted as a weight loss supplement by reducing sugar cravings. Dosage varies, and at present there is not enough scientific evidence that establishes a recommended dosage range. Gymnema tablets and capsules are also available. The most important thing to remember when purchasing nutritional supplements is the source and integrity of the manufacturer. To start, I recommend taking 250 milligrams of Gymnema three times a day.

New Hope Core Nutritional Supplements

Supplement	Contains	Daily Dosage Instructions
Digestive Enzymes Ultra	Blend of enzymes, Betaine HCL	1-2 capsules with meals
Multi-strain Probiotics	50 billion CFU's	1-2 capsules a day on empty stomach
Trace Minerals	Zinc	30-60 milligrams
	Chromium	200-400 milligrams
	Magnesium	200-300 milligrams
L-methylfolate	Folate	800 micrograms-15 milligrams
B-Complex	Vitamins B1, B3, B6	25-100 milligrams
Essential fatty acids (EFA)	Omega-3 fatty acids and omega-6 fatty acids	1-3 grams
Curcumin	Curcumin	250 milligrams-1gram
Inositol (powder)	Inositol	4-12 grams
Gymnema	Gymnema	250 milligrams three times a day

Summary

Nutrient deficiencies often contribute to the stranglehold of appetite disturbances and can intensify devastating patterns of disordered eating. Working with a qualified healthcare practitioner to identify personal nutrient imbalances and implement a unique supplementation plan can be a powerful step in recovery.

Several vitamins, minerals, and other supplements have been found to be particularly influential in appetite regulation. One such group is the B vitamins; namely, B-6, folate, and B-12, which work synergistically to provide energy, fight fatigue, neutralize sugar cravings, and prevent mood fluctuations related to hypoglycemia. In addition to its supportive role in immune function, vitamin C is also involved in appetite. This antioxidant works to improve insulin function and glucose metabolism. It is often depleted in those with high sugar diets.

Three primary minerals are associated with disrupted eating behaviors: chromium, which helps to stabilize glucose, minimize cravings, and control the symptoms of atypical depression; magnesium, which prevents insulin resistant hunger, anxiety, and depression; and zinc, which can be critical to the treatment of depression and the restoration of a normal appetite in those with anorexia. The essential fatty acids omega-3 and omega-6 must also be present in proper ratios to regulate metabolism, maintain neurotransmitter balance, and control inflammation. Inositol heightens insulin sensitivity and participates in the action of serotonin as well. Probiotics that work to bolster the friendly bacteria in the digestive tract are important in ensuring that nutrients are assimilated from foods in the first place.

When used as part of an individualized, integrative treatment plan, supplements can help to enhance metabolism, stabilize blood sugar, and resynchronize hormones, thereby restoring appetite to a helpful and harmonious normal. Taking supplements to correct nutritional deficiencies is the foundation in the New Hope model for restoring appetite control.

Key Points

- Taking certain supplements in appropriate doses, based on the results of your metabolic tests, may be of immense value in solving your appetite disturbances.

- B vitamins are important to mood and appetite regulation. B6 is especially important as it is a cofactor in serotonin synthesis.
- Inositol enhances insulin sensitivity and may be an effective treatment for depression.
- Low folate levels are linked to depression. A form called L-methylfolate may work more effectively than regular folate supplements because it can cross the blood-brain barrier.
- Chromium helps improve insulin function and may help ease depression, carbohydrate cravings, and weight gain.
- Magnesium helps fight insulin resistance and depression.
- Zinc affects hormones and peptides that regulate the appetite. Zinc deficiency is related to depression and anorexia.
- A deficiency or imbalance of essential fatty acids can contribute to depression, obesity, and diabetes, all of which can affect eating habits and appetite.
- Be sure to work with a physician or healthcare provider familiar with the concept of biochemical individuality to create a supplement program that is appropriate for you.

PART III.
MEDICATIONS FOR BINGE EATING AND FOOD ADDICTION

11
CONTROLLING APPETITE WITH MEDICATIONS

For some of you, a medication or a combination of medications can provide additional support to overcome binge eating or food addiction. This additional help is especially important when disordered eating coexists alongside emotional or psychiatric conditions like depression, anxiety, or ADHD. In Chapter 10, I discussed nutritional interventions, including a blend of all the essential amino acids that serve as precursors to neurotransmitters that control appetite. I have found amino acid supplementation is effective in breaking the cycle of disordered eating in many patients. For others, amino acids alone do not provide adequate symptomatic relief, and in such cases, medications can be extraordinarily helpful. The New Hope model is an integrative approach to treatment and might be an option to optimize neurotransmitter levels to get off the roller coaster of food addiction and binge eating.

Understanding the powerful addictive qualities of certain foods—including sugar, dairy, and gluten—will hopefully help you to appreciate the biological components of binge eating disorder and food addiction. When needed, medications can provide the biological brakes to stop disordered eating.

As discussed in Chapter 4, patients with disordered eating may have co-occurring psychiatric problems that are too often ignored or misdiagnosed. Anxiety, depression, bipolar disorder, Post-traumatic Stress Disorder (PTSD) and, perhaps most common, Attention Deficit Hyperactivity

Disorder (ADHD) complicate effective treatment for patients struggling with disordered eating. Receptors and molecules that modulate hunger and satiety are intertwined with receptors and molecules that control emotions, behavior, and cognition. Medication to treat these co-occurring problems also helps with binge eating and disordered appetite. In some cases, evidence exists from early studies to show that medications already approved by the U.S. Food and Drug Administration (FDA) to treat co-occurring psychiatric problems will help patients control disordered eating.

Suggesting medicine as a treatment for food addiction raises a red flag with many professionals. They argue that the solution to our nation's weight problems will not be found in a bottle of pills. The concern about swallowing a pill for a quick fix seems to take away the dimension of personal responsibility. Yet we have learned over the years that diets do not work and the epidemic of disordered eating grows at a staggering rate. Again, the common message from some of my colleagues is the simple advice embodied in the Nike slogan: just do it.

Disordered eating is not a simple problem and it isn't resolved by a simple solution. Many components are involved. From working with thousands of patients, I have found that the most effective treatment for food addiction and binge eating is comprised of several complementary interventions. This is why the New Hope model is founded on the principles of integrative medicine.

Most of my patients have struggled to break the stranglehold of food addiction for a long time. They have worked hard. They have suffered through failed diets, endured shame, and wrought havoc with their metabolism by bingeing and often purging. If medication can change the biochemistry that ensnares them in food addiction, why is there so much resistance on the part of professionals to use medications? Medicine is not the enemy!

Several medications have been shown to be useful in treating patients with disordered eating. Often, treatment with a combination of medications provides permanent solutions. As disordered eating is a complicated problem, it should be no surprise that sometimes a combination of medications is necessary to completely resolve symptoms. After all, most complicated chronic diseases—including heart disease, diabetes, cancer, and hypertension—respond best to a combination of medicines.

Considering the magnitude of the problem of obesity in our culture, you may be disappointed and surprised that so few medications are actually approved by the FDA to treat disordered eating. There are several reasons for this. One is the stigma associated with binge eating and obesity that still prevails in our culture. Second is the issue of profit. Early studies of existing drugs to combat obesity often showed the drugs to be ineffective in long-term studies or associated with high dropout rates. These outcomes meant delays for the pharmaceutical companies in getting a drug to market, thus minimizing their profits.

To receive FDA approval, any new drug must be evaluated in three phases. The first phase is conducted with a small group of patients. It is designed to evaluate the safety of the drug and the maximum dose that can be tolerated without significant side effects. If the drug passes this initial test, it is evaluated in a Phase II study, which involves more patients and tests both the safety and the effectiveness of the drug. Once it is judged both safe and effective, the drug may enter Phase III trials. These research studies involve large numbers of patients, often at more than one research institution. Phase III studies are designed to compare the effectiveness of a new drug against placebo or sugar pills. Once a medication has been demonstrated to be effective, it meets the criteria for FDA approval.

Some researchers now question this standard process for medication approval. Our increasing knowledge of genetic variability and biochemical individuality may prove that results from large clinical trials are not really helpful insofar as guiding treatment for individuals. Despite the time, money, and effort poured into monitoring these clinical trials, the variability between individuals can be great enough that at any given time, two patients with the same illness can be given the same drug but have completely different reactions. In a recent article published in *The New York Times*, the author Clifton Leaf raises the questions: "Do clinical trials work? Are the diseases of individuals so particular that testing experimental medicines in broad groups is doomed to create more frustration than knowledge?" Clearly, biochemical individuality complicates any general diagnostic recommendations.

The Options

When I consider adding medication to the essential biological foundation of nutritional therapy, I first consider the most commonly prescribed antidepressants, the *selective serotonin reuptake inhibitors*, or SSRIs. With professional guidance, these can be used in combination with amino acids and, if necessary, with other medications.

SSRIs

Neurotransmitters are chemical messengers in the brain that contain the keys to optimal brain functioning. The neurotransmitters—serotonin, dopamine, and norepinephrine—help brain cells communicate with each other. Of those, serotonin is most closely linked with mood, appetite, and a feeling of well-being. The SSRIs are a class of drugs that target serotonin.

The SSRIs don't actually increase serotonin production; instead, they work by increasing the amount of serotonin available in the brain. When your serotonin levels drop, you may crave sweets and starches and may even binge and purge. Serotonin imbalances are also associated with depressed mood, apathy, poor impulse control, obsessive-compulsive disorder (OCD), panic disorder, and insomnia, all of which contribute to disordered eating behaviors.

Increasing the level of serotonin available in the brain may help patients reestablish a more orderly pattern of eating. Optimizing serotonin can slow the cycle of bingeing and purging. Simultaneously, it helps mitigate the effects of coexisting depression, OCD, and anxiety.

The SSRIs include fluoxetine (Prozac), sertraline (Zoloft), fluvoxamine (Luvox), escitalopram (Lexapro) and citalopram (Celexa). Research has repeatedly demonstrated that optimal dosages for treating disordered eating with SSRIs are higher than the usual doses most physicians prescribe for depression.

Because scientists recognize that increasing serotonin may help interrupt the neural patterns underlying disordered eating, many research trials have tested the effects of various SSRIs on bulimia, binge eating disorder, and other manifestations of disordered eating.

At present, fluoxetine (Prozac) is the only medication approved by the FDA for treating an eating disorder, bulimia nervosa. The approval was based on large studies at several medical centers. These double-blinded studies involved two groups of patients. One group was given Prozac and the other was given a placebo. When the study was unblinded and the identity of who was in which group was revealed, researchers realized that the patients taking Prozac experienced much greater relief from the symptoms of bulimia than the patients taking placebo did. Another study involving eighty-five patients with binge eating disorder compared patients treated with Prozac and those given placebo. The patients on Prozac engaged in fewer binges than their counterparts on placebo.

Other research confirms these encouraging results. A review of forty-seven studies on treatments for bulimia found that 60 milligrams of Prozac per day decreases binge eating, purging and related psychological problems in the short term.

Another SSRI, Zoloft, has also been evaluated in clinical studies. Twenty patients with bulimia took part in a randomized, twelve-week study testing the effectiveness of sertraline, or Zoloft. Those patients taking Zoloft engaged in fewer episodes of bingeing and purging than those who received placebo. A second study compared the effectiveness of the two SSRIs Prozac and Zoloft. Patients with binge eating disorder in both groups lost weight and their bingeing diminished—outcomes that were maintained for the twenty-four weeks of the study. The study showed no appreciable difference in the effectiveness of the two SSRIs.

At least one study, however, has shown that the response to SSRIs may be only short term, as Prozac appeared no more effective than a placebo in reducing binge frequency or body weight after sixteen weeks of treatment. In other words, after the initial improvement on the medication, there was a gradual return to disordered eating. This is why an integrated nutritional and medication approach can be so effective in preventing symptom relapse as opposed to an approach based solely on medication.

While the SSRIs can help some patients with bulimia or binge eating, I have found that the SSRIs alone rarely lead to complete remission of binge eating or food addiction, or to sustained weight loss. If additional help is needed to achieve remission of bingeing, I often prescribe an augmenting agent. The first augmenting agent I try is a medication that was originally intended to treat seizures: topiramate, or Topamax.

Topamax

Researchers first realized the potential of Topamax (topiramate) as a treatment for binge eating disorder when epilepsy studies showed that patients not only achieved relief from seizures but also experienced a decrease in appetite and lost weight. This discovery led to research exploring the effects of Topamax on binge eating, bulimia, and obesity. The results of several independent studies were strikingly positive. A clinical trial conducted at the University of Florida in 2000 explored the effects of Topamax on thirteen women with binge eating disorder plus depression, anxiety, ADHD, or another psychiatric problem. Nine of the thirteen patients experienced a moderate or better-than-moderate improvement, which continued from three to thirty months. The patients also lost weight; seven of them lost more than eleven pounds.

Many patients have tried using *cognitive-behavioral therapy* (CBT) to identify and address underlying factors of their disordered eating behavior. CBT, which acknowledges that certain behaviors cannot be controlled by rational thought, will be discussed in more detail in Chapter 15. CBT in conjunction with medications may be helpful for many of you. One study assessed the effects of Topamax and CBT on disordered eating. This randomized, double-blind, placebo-controlled trial involved seventy-three overweight patients. The patients received CBT plus either 200 milligrams of Topamax or a placebo for twenty-one weeks. The patient group taking

Topamax lost an average of fifteen pounds during the study, compared to an average two-pound weight loss for those in the placebo group. Furthermore, eighty-four percent of patients in the Topamax group were able to stop bingeing.

Interestingly, combining Topamax with CBT improved the efficacy of each approach. This conclusion is important because, although CBT has been consistently shown to be the most effective psychotherapy for patients with disordered eating, CBT alone is more effective in the short term than in the long term. CBT helps patients identify distorted thinking about themselves and about food, and shows them better ways to cope with stress. Therapy may break the cycle of distorted eating for some, but medications may still be necessary in order to address underlying neurobiological disturbances. This study showed how helpful Topamax can be to sustain the positive effects from CBT.

Further research has confirmed encouraging results from treatment with Topamax. In another randomized, double-blind, placebo-controlled study lasting fourteen weeks, Topamax reduced binge frequency by ninety-four percent, compared to a reduction of forty-six percent in the patients taking placebo. Topamax also resulted in significant reductions in patients' body mass index, weight, and symptom severity.

A review of five clinical trials examining the effects of Topamax on bulimia and binge eating disorder, published in 2008, decisively determined that the medication outperformed a placebo. On Topamax, people binged less often, ate less during binges, and lost weight.

A recent overview of several research studies of the effectiveness of Topamax in managing eating disorders concluded that Topamax reduces binge eating and night eating in overweight patients. Topamax affects not only weight and appetite but also the neural systems involved in regulating appetite to achieve hunger management.

Zonisamide

Once researchers realized the potential of Topamax for reducing obesity and sustaining healthier eating habits, they started to study additional anti-convulsion medications. In early studies, zonisamide has shown potential as part of our armamentarium of anti-obesity drugs. Zonisamide is a sulfa drug originally intended to treat seizures, but it shows promise for treating binge eating disorder and food addiction because it works by increasing levels of serotonin and dopamine in the brain.

Research proves that zonisamide helps reduce symptoms of disordered eating. Study results published in *Psychiatry* in 2009 compared the effectiveness of treatment with cognitive-based therapy alone versus CBT in conjunction with zonisamide. The study concluded that patients who received both CBT and zonisamide lost more weight, had fewer binge episodes, and displayed fewer symptoms of depression and anxiety than those who received CBT alone.

Zonisamide may also decrease the likelihood of *nonsuicidal self-injury* (NSSI). In one study, seventeen women with either bulimia or binge eating disorder received zonisamide in addition to their previously prescribed medications. While the participant numbers were small, the research suggested that zonisamide helped prevent NSSI behavior in patients with co-occurring disordered eating. Since disordered eating is often linked with self-harm, this is an important finding.

Several studies have shown that zonisamide helps reduce binge eating and thereby leads to weight loss. In most of these clinical trials, however, several patients withdrew because of unpleasant side effects. The most prevalent side effects include altered taste, fatigue, dry mouth, insomnia, indigestion, and drowsiness.

Topamax appears to have the greatest potential for treating binge eating. Topamax is able to suppress the underlying causes of weight gain and to diminish the biological counter-response that results from weight loss. There are many research studies supporting its use, and I have seen time and again how Topamax helps patients achieve success in overcoming cravings and the inability to stop binge eating. For many patients, Topamax has provided the biological break from the brain's habitual circuitry.

In my practice I have rarely seen a problem with side effects of Topamax. An occasional patient has a mild problem feeling sedated until the dosage is adjusted. The Internet is filled with stories of Topamax side effects, primarily sedation and memory problems. Some bloggers have called it "Dopamax", suggesting that the medicine makes you dopey. In most patients, side effects of Topamax occur only in higher doses (200–400 milligrams) than I typically prescribe for binge eating. I have found low doses (25–200 milligrams) effective without causing side effects. Other side effects include numbness and tingling in the arms and legs, fatigue, changes in taste, and gastrointestinal distress. As with any medication, you should report any side effects to your physician.

One patient whose life had long been dominated by disordered eating finally found success when I prescribed this medication. She left a message on my answering machine: "God bless Topamax!"

Stimulants

The standard treatment for Attention Deficit Hyperactivity Disorder (ADHD) involves stimulant medications. *Stimulants* are a class of medications that have been used since 1938 for the treatment of attention deficits and hyperactivity. As discussed in Chapter 4, many patients with disordered eating are often undiagnosed or never treated for coexisting disorders such as ADHD.

One stimulant that can augment treatment for disordered eating is phentermine. Originally approved more than fifty years ago for treating obesity, it works by mimicking the appetite-suppressing effects of norepinephrine in the brain. Phentermine was the "Phen" part of Fen Phen, a wildly popular diet drug in the 1990s that was taken off the market when fenfluramine (the "fen" part) was implicated in dangerous side effects, including hypertension and heart valve problems.

Although phentermine by itself is still in use, a new medication has shown even more promise for treatment of obesity. By combining a very low dose of phentermine with a low dose of Topamax, researchers have produced a medication called Qsymia. This medication, approved by the FDA in early 2012 to treat obesity, has already helped many patients interrupt binge eating, lose weight, and improve their blood pressure and cholesterol.

A research study called "CONQUER" yielded promising results. This fifty-six-week trial enrolled 2,487 overweight adults and randomly assigned them to receive either a placebo or one of two doses of the combination of phentermine and Topamax: a lower dose and a higher dose. The participants in the placebo group lost an average of three pounds, while those in the lower dose medication group lost an average of eighteen pounds. Those taking the higher dose of phentermine plus Topamax lost an average of twenty-two pounds. Improvements in metabolic risk factors were observed in both medication groups, but not in the placebo group.

A follow-up to the CONQUER study continued with the same group of participants for another fifty-six weeks to study longer term effects of the phentermine and Topamax combination. Researchers found the medication combination continued to produce significant weight loss even after two years. The placebo group lost an average of 1.8% of their body weight over the entire 108 weeks of the study, while the low-dose medication group lost an average of nine percent. The high-dose medication group lost an average of twenty percent of their body weight. Moreover, most patients had no trouble with side effects over the course of 108 weeks.

I frequently prescribe Topamax and stimulant medications together but prefer for patients to take them as separate medications rather than a combination pill. This allows for adjustments to be made to both medications more easily.

A medication approved for the treatment of ADHD, Vyvanse, also shows promise for treating binge eating. Phase II of the clinical trial evaluating Vyvanse was completed in 2012; Phase III yielded preliminary positive results in November 2013. And, as of February of 2015, Vyvanse was granted approval by the FDA for the treatment of binge eating disorder.

Integrative Medicine for Binge Eating

The Phase II study was a randomized, double-blind, placebo-controlled study that included 213 patients diagnosed with moderate to severe binge eating disorder. Patients' daily food intake and binge history were monitored for eleven weeks. Patients were divided into four groups: the first received the placebo, the second a dose of 30 milligrams of Vyvanse daily, the third a daily dose of 50 milligrams, and the fourth 70 milligrams of Vyvanse per day.

Researchers observed differences in the number and frequency of binge episodes. The patients on 50 milligrams experienced a decrease in bingeing from 4.540 to 0.310 days per week. Taking 70 milligrams of Vyvanse, patients' binge frequency decreased from 4.470 to 0.011 after the trial. The most dramatic difference: a total elimination of binge episodes for one entire week, a benchmark achieved by week eleven of the trial. Sixty-seven percent of patients in the group taking 70 milligrams of Vyvanse were free from bingeing for the last week, compared to fifty-six of patients on the 50 milligrams dose and thirty-four percent of patients on the placebo.

Phase III studies had an enrollment of 773 patients ages eighteen to fifty-five with moderate to severe binge eating disorder. Patients were randomized to Vyvanse or placebo treatment groups, and all Vyvanse-treated patients began at a dose of 30 milligrams before the dose was increased to either 50 or 70 milligrams. In both of these studies, Vyvanse was found to be more effective than the placebo in reducing the number of binge days per week.

Stimulant medications increase the availability of the neurotransmitter dopamine. We know that enhancing dopamine production can play an important role in regulating the binge eating cycle and curbing food addiction. I have seen in my practice that when I prescribe a stimulant drug to treat ADHD, it also helps to blunt the cravings and lack of impulse control that underlie binge eating.

Like many medications, stimulants can be abused. Some patients with eating disorders have used stimulants to help restrict their eating in an unhealthy way. In my experience, patients with binge eating disorder do not tend to abuse these medications. Instead, these patients find considerable gratification and improved self-esteem through finally being able to control the desire to binge and obtaining relief from long-untreated symptoms of ADHD.

Naltrexone

For patients who continue to experience disordered eating that is not sufficiently helped by SSRIs, Topamax, stimulants or some combination of these, I often prescribe naltrexone, an opioid antagonist. Naltrexone is a medication used to reduce the cravings associated with alcohol addiction. It also works well for many patients with out-of-control eating behaviors such as binge eating or bingeing and purging.

Like any other addiction, disordered eating involves complicated neurocircuitry in the brain with effects that often require pharmacological intervention to break the cycle of craving. It surprises me that the neurobiology of addiction is rarely addressed in treatment for eating disorders. I have found that treating the addiction is often the key to recovery.

At the root of the neurochemistry of addiction is the rush of *endorphins* that becomes the driver of cravings. These hormone-like chemicals that are naturally produced by the brain and induce a sense of well-being. They dull the sensation of pain, produce feelings of euphoria, promote the release of sex hormones, enhance the immune response, and modulate appetite. Endorphins reinforce behaviors such as eating, having sex, cuddling babies, and exercising. Unfortunately, they also reinforce potentially destructive behaviors such as drinking alcohol, bingeing, purging, and gambling. Engaging in any of these behaviors also leads to a flood of endorphins in the brain.

Behaviors that lead to an endorphin rush are learned and then reinforced by the reward of feelings of pleasure and contentment. When you drink alcohol, endorphins are released. You drink again to re-experience this sense of pleasure.

Just as these behaviors can be learned, they can also be unlearned. Naltrexone is a medication that acts as an opiate antagonist. If you take naltrexone before drinking, endorphins are still released, but the naltrexone prevents them from binding to cell receptors.

Naltrexone helps stop destructive addictive behaviors by removing the endorphin reward. It blocks opioid receptors that bind to endorphins, thereby regulating the pleasure response. Endorphins are like ships that must dock before they can unload their goods. In this case the dock is the opioid receptor and the goods are the pleasurable feelings. By making it impossible for the endorphins to dock, naltrexone takes away the endorphin rush. The endorphins yield no effect. Over time, the nervous system slowly weakens the neural connections that cause cravings and addictive behavior.

Analysis of many clinical trials supports the use of naltrexone in the treatment of alcoholism. There is strong evidence that naltrexone significantly reduces alcohol relapses in individuals struggling with alcohol addiction.

One approach utilizing naltrexone in the treatment of alcohol addiction is referred to as the *Sinclair method*. This method is not based on abstinence; instead, patients are encouraged to take naltrexone before drinking. They no longer experience the pleasure they formerly associated with drinking, and their cravings and drinking gradually decrease over a period of months. If, for instance, alcohol no longer produced intense cravings, your brain would eventually reprogram itself. Behaviors once learned would be unlearned through the mechanism called *pharmacological extinction*. After a while, although you might still enjoy alcohol, you would not be driven by uncontrollable urges and cravings to consume excess alcohol.

The Sinclair method, as studied in various scientific papers, has led to striking reductions in alcohol addiction, especially in the Scandinavian countries, where it was introduced. The use of naltrexone for treating alcoholism is also well-established by scientific research in the USA.

Like alcohol abuse, binge eating for some is driven by cravings for endorphins. A blast of endorphins can be a powerful - but temporary - fix for depression, anxiety, stress, or lack of energy. The bulimic cycle releases endorphins, especially the purging phase, which in itself can become addictive even when bingeing isn't present. These bingeing and purging behaviors are repeated to achieve an endorphin rush that temporarily dulls emotional and physical pain. Research exploring alcohol addiction helps clarify the mechanisms behind food addiction. Much of the treatment success with alcoholism has occurred in programs based on abstinence. For obvious reasons, these approaches are not transferrable to food addiction treatment, since one cannot abstain from food. Fortunately, the Sinclair method, which is not predicated on abstinence, is also applicable when the substance fueling cravings is food.

I have seen great success using naltrexone. Not only does it interfere with the reinforcement of disordered eating, it also increases endorphin levels the following day, helping to prevent or lessen these behaviors. For disordered eating that is not relieved by SSRIs, Topamax, or stimulants, I often initially prescribe 25–50 milligrams of naltrexone to be taken at times the patient feels likely to be vulnerable to bingeing. The combination of naltrexone and amino acids is a powerful tool to help patients extinguish food addiction and get off the roller coaster.

I have seen few side effects from low-dose naltrexone. For some patients, higher doses are necessary to curb food addiction. With 100–200 milligrams, gastrointestinal upsets such as diarrhea may occur. When taken at higher than recommended doses (300 milligrams), some reports of liver damage have been documented. Therefore, liver function tests should be conducted prior to beginning treatment with naltrexone and periodically thereafter.

A recent study in Finland administered the drug *naloxone* to patients in the form of a nasal spray. Naloxone has the same pharmacological effects as naltrexone, but it is shorter-acting. A total of 127 overweight women participated in this Phase II study over twenty-four weeks. The participants were able to reduce their binge eating by seventy-five percent during this period.

Medication Combinations

Medications and, often, combinations of medications utilized in a systematic way based upon symptoms, coexisting psychiatric disorders, and genetics can provide permanent relief from lifelong patterns of disordered eating. Combinations of medications have sometimes unlocked the door for treating obesity and binge eating, which were once resistant to trials with individual drugs. Combinations of medications can often be more beneficial than single medications. First, lower dosages of each can be administered, minimizing the potential for side effects and adverse reactions. Moreover, combinations affect different neurocircuitries in the brain to help patients sustain positive results with less chance of relapse.

One useful combination for binge eating is the SSRIs in combination with naltrexone. The combination of the SSRI fluoxetine and naltrexone has been shown to be effective in treating heroin addiction. Naltrexone and fluoxetine have also been shown to be a promising combination for treating disordered eating. When naltrexone is combined with fluoxetine, it appears be effective at a reduced dose. In one study, four patients received naltrexone alone, fluoxetine alone and, finally, a combination of the two over a twelve-week period. The patients responded most favorably to the drug combination, and all of them experienced a striking decrease in binges. In another study, a patient taking fluoxetine with 100 milligrams of naltrexone daily found great relief from the craving to binge, and her weight declined from 57 to 49 kg. Italian researchers showed that several bulimic patients taking a combination of fluoxetine and naltrexone successfully resolved their disordered eating.

Many medications, including promising medication combinations, are now available to help patients get off the roller coaster and end the cycle of food addiction. I consider medication not as a quick fix, but as one strategy to help patients reclaim a healthy relationship with food. I believe it is important to go beyond black-and-white thinking—not to claim that there is one true solution to the problem of disordered eating, but rather to acknowledge that many interventions can contribute to success.

James Greenblatt, MD

In the book *Brain over Binge*, the author Kathryn Hansen documents her own success in getting off the food addiction roller coaster. Through most of the book she attributes her success exclusively to willpower. The book concludes, "After 6 years of chronic bingeing and purging, Kathryn stopped her eating disorder independently and abruptly using one tool and one tool only: the power of her own brain."

This description makes her solution sound very simple. But at one place tucked away in the middle pages of the book, the author acknowledges that something else helped her:

> "I was fortunate to have the experience with the medication Topamax that temporarily alleviated my urges to binge. Nearly 2 years prior to my recovery, Topamax taught me that the problem wasn't my life or my inability to cope with it. It also taught me that, without urges to binge, I didn't need the secondary benefits of binge eating—nor did I want them. When my urges to binge temporarily subsided while on the drug, I didn't feel the need to be sugar-drunk: I didn't feel a need to be temporarily numb to my problems: I didn't feel a need for the pleasure that binge eating brought me."

Hansen's book, like so much of the literature from the eating disorder community, proclaims that willpower alone can defeat food addiction. Yet the author's own experience is actually a powerful testament to the value of Topamax in loosening the grip of binge eating and food addiction!

Research into medications to treat disordered eating is still in its early stages. Only one medication has been approved by the FDA to treat most types of disordered eating. Many of the medication study results now available have limitations, including small sample size and a sole focus on one medication only. In addition, with the exception of obesity and major depressive disorder, there has been no large scientific study of medication results in patients with food addiction and co-occurring psychiatric conditions. We need studies conducted on combinations of drugs—for instance,

Topamax together with SSRIs—as a basis to help determine optimal treatment regimens for individual patients.

Because of biochemical individuality, it sometimes takes a medication trial to find the optimal medication therapy for an individual patient's disordered eating. The complete nutritional testing patients have already undergone helps provide a safeguard against potential side effects. While individual drugs may have limited effectiveness as sole agents, combining them with another medication can dramatically increase their efficacy. These combinations can help sustain relief from binge eating and support weight loss in patients who have been unable to maintain improvements and have relapsed.

Although research into the effectiveness of medication combinations is in its early stages, I have seen successful outcomes in patients for whom I have prescribed such a combination. In many cases, the results are astonishing. Women and men have reported freedom from compulsions to binge, and elation over weight loss that they had previously believed impossible to achieve or maintain. According to the New Hope model, medications can be a helpful and, sometimes, essential part of treatment for some people. In tandem with therapy and nutritional supplements, medications may be the critical component of an integrative intervention to end the roller-coaster ride of disordered eating.

> **DISCLAIMER:** Prior to medication being approved for use in patients in the United States, the Federal Drug Administration (FDA) mandates the drug be tested in humans in clinical research trials. Each trial looks at one or more specific areas where the drug must prove itself to be effective. For each area of effectiveness that is studied and proven, the manufacturer receives an "approved medication" for which the drug can be marketed and sold. Commonly medications appear to be effective and are often ultimately studied and proven to be effective for conditions other than the original "approved medication(s)." This is where a physician discusses their experience in using a specific drug for a non-FDA-approved

medication indication including its effectiveness and safety. The medications discussed in this book are not FDA approved for the treatment of binge eating disorder.

Summary

Supplements and targeted nutritional changes are very powerful tools for breaking the cycle of food addiction and normalizing appetite. However, in some individuals these approaches simply aren't enough to reset the disrupted biological patterning at the root of disordered eating habits. In such cases, carefully prescribed medication can provide a safe and effective biochemical solution. Several classes of medications have been found useful in treating disordered eating, with each working through a unique mechanism in the body.

The SSRIs, such as Prozac and Zoloft, block the uptake of serotonin and increase its availability within the brain, thereby minimizing symptoms of craving and anxiety often associated with bingeing. Selected anticonvulsants, including the well-studied medication Topamax, have proven useful in stabilizing the neural systems involved in weight control and appetite. Stimulant medications like Vyvanse and Phentermine can also be helpful in increasing dopamine levels and normalizing sporadic eating habits, especially in patients who struggle with an underlying diagnosis of ADHD. Naltrexone can be used to block the opioid surge that occurs with eating and reduce addictive cravings associated with food.

Although medication is not a simple fix for disordered eating, it can provide valuable biological support as part of an integrative plan to restore normal eating and a healthier relationship with food.

Key Points

- When nutritional interventions and supplementation do not provide adequate support, medications can be helpful

in augmenting treatment for patients struggling with disordered eating.
- An individualized combination of medications proves most effective in stopping the roller coaster of disordered eating.
- SSRIs such as Prozac and Zoloft help decrease cravings and anxiety associated with bingeing and purging by blocking the reuptake of serotonin and increasing its availability in the brain.
- Topamax, an anticonvulsant medication, helps normalize the neural systems involved in appetite regulation and weight control.
- Zonisamide has shown promise in treating binge eating disorder and food addiction by increasing the neurotransmitters serotonin and dopamine in the brain.
- Stimulants can be useful for disordered eating patients struggling with an underlying diagnosis of ADHD.
- For patients who do not respond to SSRIs, Topamax or stimulants, the opioid antagonist naltrexone can help to reduce the addictive cravings associated with foods.
- Medications do not offer an easy or immediate fix to disordered eating, but they can be used as part of an integrative approach to rebuild a healthy relationship with food.

PART IV.
LIFESTYLE CHANGES FOR BINGE EATING AND FOOD ADDICTION

12
WHAT NOT TO EAT: HIGH FRUCTOSE CORN SYRUP & ARTIFICIAL SWEETENERS

Perhaps you are in the process of exploring whether medication can help with appetite control, and you have identified which supplements and amino acids you need to adjust your metabolism. These approaches involve taking in substances to help normalize your biochemistry and control your appetite. Integrative medicine, the field on which this book is based, also calls for a third approach. This approach consists of lifestyle changes you can make to help you get off the roller coaster and reclaim not only a healthy appetite but a fulfilling life as well.

In the following chapters, I will review some dietary guidelines to help address food addiction and binge eating. These guidelines are not part of another "diet" for rapid weight loss but are instead meant to provide you with information about how certain components in foods can contribute to or exacerbate food addiction. The goal is to avoid these foods to improve overall health, and to provide an easier journey off the roller coaster of disordered eating.

As we have discussed in the previous chapters, certain components in food, such as sugar, casomorphin, and gliadorphin, can affect the mind and body in ways analogous to opiate drugs like heroin and morphine.

Some foods are especially likely to trigger an addictive process. Sugar is particularly dangerous not only because of its addictive-like properties, but also because it acts as a nutritional vacuum. When we consume sugar, B vitamins are used to metabolize it, stripping us of much-needed B vitamins necessary for other important functions such as neurotransmitter synthesis. Knowing the damage sugar can cause, what compels us to eat more of it? Researchers at Stony Brook University identified a sweet spot of the brain that operates in an irregular way when simple sugars are given to people with insulin resistance. People with this metabolic syndrome exhibited a slower release of dopamine in a major pleasure center of the brain. The decreased dopamine release suggests that insulin-resistant individuals may be facing a deficient reward system, which leads them to consume more sugar in order to feel the pleasurable effects of consuming sugar. This sets off the roller-coaster ride and the cycle of disordered eating.

I have discussed sugar as the basis of food addiction in Chapter 6. In this chapter, I want to discuss the most commonly utilized form of sugar in processed foods: high fructose corn syrup.

Alcohol without the Buzz: High Fructose Corn Syrup

High fructose corn syrup (HFCS) is made from corn that is spun at a high velocity and combined with three different enzymes to create thick, super-sweet syrup. Dr. Robert Lustig, the former chairman of the Obesity Task Force of the Pediatric Endocrine Society, has declared that HFCS "should be considered alcohol without the buzz." Just like alcohol, the more HFCS you consume, the more likely you are to develop an addiction—a craving for more food, an inability to stop eating, a preoccupation with the next meal, and withdrawal symptoms when you stop.

High fructose corn syrup should be avoided if you are trying to step off the roller coaster of food addiction. Unfortunately, that is not an easy task: HFCS is *everywhere*. It now comprises more than forty percent of caloric sweeteners added to food and beverages and is the major caloric sweetener in soft drinks manufactured in the United States. It is replacing sugar in baked goods, cereals, canned fruits, jellies, dairy desserts, and flavored yogurt. HCFS is now even used in foods that don't have a sweet taste, including chowders and processed meats such as sausage and ham. With HFCS in so many foods and drinks, it is not surprising that Americans now consume an average of twelve teaspoons of HFCS *per day*, with teenagers consuming eighty percent more than the national average.

Why is HFCS so prevalent? First, it is inexpensive, costing only half the price of sugar. Second, only a small amount of HFCS is needed to infuse food with intense sweetness. Companies therefore find it cost-effective to use a small quantity of HFCS instead of a larger amount of a more expensive sweetener or flavor. Third, HFCS also works as a preservative, so it prolongs shelf life and gives food a moist, chewy consistency. It is also easy to transport. All these attributes make HFCS the ideal choice among people whose job it is to manufacture and sell food.

Dangers of High Fructose Corn Syrup

Why exactly is HFCS dangerous? Several reasons. Through the process of metabolism, HFCS is converted primarily into fat and triglycerides. One research study showed that people who ate HFCS-sweetened food had two hundred percent higher levels of triglycerides than those who consumed food sweetened with glucose. Elevated triglyceride levels are linked with cardiovascular problems. The body also has a much more difficult time breaking HFCS down than sugar, a difficulty which over time causes weight gain. Body fat from HFCS tends to accumulate around the abdomen, a pattern of weight gain that increases the risk of cardiovascular disease more than other weight gain patterns. Disturbing as this is, it's far from the end of the story when it comes to the health dangers of HFCS. HFCS is metabolized in the liver, where it causes insulin resistance that can hasten the development of diabetes. HFCS also often contains the toxic element mercury. One research study found that almost half of tested samples of food containing HFCS, particularly where the substance was listed among the top ingredients, were contaminated with mercury.

Most relevant to its addictive properties, consumption of HFCS leads to *leptin resistance*. As we have discussed elsewhere in this book, the chemical messages sent by the hormone leptin are very important for weight control, regulating the balance between energy expenditure and food intake. Leptin signals the hypothalamus in the brain how much fat to store. The more fat the body stores, the more leptin is released, signaling a sense of fullness that, in turn, sends the message to the body that food intake can be curtailed and calories should be burned off. When HFCS is consumed, however, leptin receptors become desensitized, so the hypothalamus does not get the signal it should. Instead of feeling full, the person can't stop eating, finds it difficult to control cravings, and gains weight.

The relationship between HFCS and leptin resistance is very clear in research animals. One group of scientists demonstrated that rats given a diet of HFCS developed leptin resistance even before their body weight changed; this was the first signal that their body weight would eventually spiral out of control. Moreover, those rats that developed leptin resistance went on to gain more weight and become overweight more rapidly in response to a high-fat diet—even when they were no longer fed HFCS. This tendency to store more fat more quickly appeared to arise solely from chronic HFCS consumption. According to University of Florida researcher Philip J. Scarpace, the HFCS did its damage by "fooling the brain so that it ignores leptin."

The weight gain in these rats on a diet of HFCS was astounding. The rats gained significantly more weight than those with access to table sugar even when they ate the same overall number of calories. And the remarkable weight gain did not occur only in a small group of rats. When rats are fed a high-fat diet, some gain extra weight, but others do not. A Princeton research team demonstrated that when rats drink HFCS at levels even well below those found in soda pop, they become overweight—*every single one.*

The Princeton team concluded that rats become addicted to HFCS, causing effects in the brain similar to those caused by drugs of abuse. Other researchers also marvel at the powerful effect of this sweetener on rats. Scripps Institute researchers found that rats fed fast food containing HFCS are willing to withstand electric shocks to their feet and cold temperatures in order to get more HFCS.

In most mammals, sweet receptors evolved in ancestral environments that were low in sugar. These receptors are not adapted to high concentrations of sweetness, so when we consume intense sweetness, our bodies generate a supranormal reward that leads to addiction along the same receptor pathways as other addictions. When the government ordered Coca-Cola to remove cocaine from its soda in the early 1900s, it was eventually replaced with HFCS. One addictive substance was simply substituted for another.

Dr. Richard Johnson, in his well-written book *The Fat Switch*, describes how the sugar *fructose* activates a metabolic change in our bodies that preferentially turns the food we eat into fat. An increase in food intake and decrease in physical activity results from activating this "switch." This is a physiological mechanism whereby fructose ingestion creates a cascade of chemical reactions that result in energy from food being preferentially converted to fat and the development of insulin resistance.

As we have already discussed, fructose is *not* similar to glucose in terms of its effect on human metabolism. When glucose is metabolized, cells remain healthy and the sugar is burned to produce energy in the form of ATP. When fructose is metabolized, there is a decrease in energy and ATP levels plummet. Apparently, the enzyme *fructokinase* needed to metabolize fructose consumes ATP in the process. This loss of energy occurs rapidly, and the process of using more energy to metabolize fructose results in the decrease of energy used for burning calories, which leads to insulin resistance.

Since fructose and glucose produce the same number of calories per gram (four calories), Dr. Johnson provides clear scientific evidence that fructose stimulates appetite and fat accumulation by a unique mechanism not found with metabolism of other sugars.

High fructose corn syrup creates metabolic chaos in every aspect of appetite and weight management. Dopamine is released with repeated consumption, inducing the pleasure response. Repeated consumption then can lead to food addiction and binge eating.

The clear-cut scientific findings of the damaging properties of HFCS have led to an outcry among professionals in the nutrition and public health communities. This outcry in turn has garnered responses from the fast-food industry, many prominent members of which have launched initiatives to drop HFCS from menus and ingredient lists.

Eliminating HFCS should be part of your treatment program. It is important to pay attention to what you eat by learning to read nutritional labels correctly. Avoid focusing on caloric content and instead learn how to read the ingredient list. Labels listing high fructose corn syrup as one of the product's first ingredients should be a warning sign to avoid this food product. As mentioned earlier, even foods that aren't considered to be sweet may still contain high fructose corn syrup. If sugar must be used, look instead for other natural sweeteners, such as pure honey, that are less harmful to your body and have a lower glycemic index than HFCS.

Artificial Sweeteners: No Magic Bullet

Since the development of the first artificial sweetener in the late 1800s, these chemically produced, nonnutritive additives that make foods taste sweeter have become staples in the diets of people around the world. Here in the US, there are presently five FDA-approved artificial sweeteners on the market—aspartame, saccharin, sucralose, acesulfame-K, and neotame—which are used to sweeten food products from baked goods and jellies to chewing gum and diet sodas. These nonnutritive additives are marketed as a convenient way to add sweetness to foods without negatively impacting blood sugar levels in diabetics or adding extra calories that could lead to weight gain. While artificial sweeteners appear to be a simple and effective sugar alternative for diabetics and a way to lower caloric intake, they do just the *opposite*.

Several studies have explored the health effects of drinking artificially sweetened diet soda. Results from one study suggest that regular consumption of diet soda can actually interfere with the body's ability to regulate blood sugar levels and weight, leading to weight gain and an increased risk of diabetes, high blood pressure, and cardiovascular problems. Another study concluded that people who consume diet sodas have a sixty-seven percent greater likelihood of developing diabetes than those who do not. The sweet taste of artificial sweeteners tricks the body into believing it that has ingested glucose, which leads to the release of insulin into the bloodstream. This insulin stores glucose as fat and lowers blood sugar, which triggers increased food intake. Because the body is not responding to its natural hunger and satiety signals, this increase in food intake can eventually lead to weight gain.

Other studies have attributed similar effects on weight to the consumption of artificial sweeteners. In a 2012 study, researchers E. Green and C. Murphy found that because these nonnutritive food additives lack calories, the body learns to no longer associate sweetness with calories and, therefore, decreases its rate of metabolism of sweet foods. This metabolic alteration, paired with the desensitization to sweetness caused by the artificial sweeteners, is associated with weight gain. It is unsurprising that research demonstrates a correlation between spikes in global obesity rates and the increased global usage of artificial sweeteners.

The effects of artificial sweeteners on weight and blood sugar levels are wholly undesirable; as with HFCS, however, the adverse effects story does not end here. In 1984, the FDA received such a high number of consumer complaints reporting problems about aspartame that they called in the Centers for Disease Control (CDC) to assist them in reviewing and evaluating the complaints. The ensuing review showed that consumers en masse reported a wide variety of negative symptoms stemming from aspartame use, ranging from neurologic and behavioral symptoms such as headaches, dizziness, and mood alterations to gastrointestinal, dermatologic, and menstrual symptoms. While artificial sweeteners may seem like an attractive option for those seeking to control weight and appetite, clearly, these nonnutritive additives may have an opposite effect.

Soft drink carbonation is also a factor contributing to weight and binge eating behaviors. The carbonation in soft drinks makes it difficult for the brain to distinguish between artificial sweeteners and sugar. When people were given an artificially-sweetened or naturally-sweetened carbonated beverage as part of a research study, the presence of carbonation reduced the degree of satiety that they experienced from the sweet taste. This may explain why some people need to drink more than one soda in order to feel satisfied.

Refined sugar and HFCS have been implicated in food addiction because their intense sweetness elicits a dopamine rush in the brain that triggers cravings for more. Over time, larger quantities of foods containing refined sugar and HFCS are required to produce the same effect, leading to binge eating behaviors. These substances also wreak havoc on your metabolism, causing wild blood sugar fluctuations and resistance to the hormones that regulate weight and food intake, leading to weight gain, diabetes, and other health problems. Artificial sweeteners were developed to avoid the negative consequences associated with refined sugar and HFCS; however, studies show that they, in fact, have the very same negative consequences. Moreover, they cause other physical ailments not associated with the ingestion of refined sugar and HFCS. Limiting your intake of refined sugar, HFCS, and artificial sweeteners can help curb your addiction to food and restore metabolic and physical health.

Summary

Certain components in food such as sugar, casomorphin, and gliadorphin can be harmful by triggering bingeing behavior and a dysregulated appetite. One of the biggest offenders is the most commonly utilized form of sugar in our processed foods: high fructose corn syrup (HFCS). Studies have shown that HFCS has addiction-triggering properties similar to opiate drugs like heroin and morphine, which makes it difficult for those who consume it regularly to stop.

While people around the world who eat westernized diets consume up to twelve teaspoons of HFCS per day, the majority are unaware of how hazardous it can be to health. HFCS consumption leads to leptin resistance, which causes leptin receptors to become so desensitized that they cannot signal the brain to stop. Animal studies have also demonstrated a clear association between HFCS consumption and weight gain. When rats drank HFCS even at levels below what we would normally find in our soda pop, every rat in the studies became obese.

HFCS creates metabolic chaos in both appetite and hunger management. Because it is concentrated and overly sweet, our reward pathways become overstimulated as we continue to consume more of it. This intense rush of dopamine triggers cravings for more. One of the first steps to take in order to regain control over your disordered eating is to eliminate foods that interfere with your body's ability to regulate appetite. It is important for consumers to be vigilant about ingredient labels listing HFCS as an ingredient and to instead seek natural alternatives.

Artificial sweeteners are laboratory-produced substances that have been manufactured and marketed as non-nutritive, low-calorie alternatives to HFCS. However, these chemical sweeteners have been found to be as damaging as their refined sugar precursors in terms of weight gain, addictive patterns, hormone dysregulation, and metabolic ruin. In addition, frequent use of artificial sweeteners can create a host of concerning physical, neurologic, and behavioral symptoms ranging from gastrointestinal upset to mood alterations. Eliminating HFCS-containing foods, decreasing use of refined sugars, and avoiding artificial sweeteners are important steps in bringing appetite back into control, and in rebuilding a stable relationship to food.

Key Points

- Sugar is a nutritional vacuum that strips your body of B vitamins that are required for brain functioning.
- Because sugar can be at the heart of food addiction, avoiding it can aid in recovery.
- High fructose corn syrup is an intense sweetener that has addictive properties as well and can lead to obesity.
- Read food labels so you can avoid foods containing high fructose corn syrup.
- Artificial sweeteners are several hundred times sweeter than sugar and cause blood sugar fluctuations that can lead to obesity and type 2 diabetes.
- Artificial sweeteners do not help people lose weight.

13
WHAT NOT TO EAT: MONOSODIUM GLUTAMATE

Another group of foods to avoid are those containing *monosodium glutamate* (MSG), a food additive that increases the palatability of foods. MSG was widely used in the United States after World War II when the US military discovered that Japanese rations tasted better than American rations. Today, food manufacturers incorporate MSG into many of their food products, since MSG restores flavor that is lost when oils are extracted. Despite its ubiquity and seemingly innocuous ability to make food taste better, MSG has powerful effects on appetite and food cravings.

Why do food manufacturers add MSG to their products? Simply because MSG improves the taste of food, stimulates a consumer's desire to eat more, and is very cheap. For example, processed food and frozen foods taste fresher and smell better if MSG is an ingredient. MSG improves the flavor of processed salad dressings and makes canned food taste less 'tinny.' Food producers can save money by omitting or cutting down on "real" ingredients and instead adding flavor "enhancers" such as MSG. Although MSG is not exactly a household word, it is now widely considered one of the five basic tastes along with sweet, sour, salty, and bitter. The flavor of MSG itself is called *umami*, which is Japanese for "delicious taste." Umami leads to a mouthwatering, satisfying sensation. It balances out the total flavor of food, making it seem more palatable. People sometimes use the word "savory" to describe umami, as the flavor is associated with rich stews and meats and other foods containing protein. Umami makes people believe that the food they are eating is more satisfying and contains more protein than it actually does. Our taste buds and brains are fooled into overestimating the quality of food prepared with MSG.

When I was in high school, my friend's family owned a Chinese restaurant. He told me the story of a customer who came into his restaurant just prior to lunchtime looking for scrambled eggs because he hadn't had breakfast. The restaurant didn't have them on the menu, but he pleaded for them to scramble him some eggs and they obliged. This man described the eggs as the best he'd ever eaten in his life, and he returned regularly thereafter for years just to eat the delectable eggs.

The reality is that as the restaurant's chef cooked the eggs, he added a huge heaping spoonful of MSG, which enhanced the flavor as well as the addictive quality of these "scrambled eggs."

Research has demonstrated that foods containing MSG make people want to eat more. Scientist John Prescott proved in several studies that food with added MSG is tastier and more appealing than food without it, and that MSG accelerates the rate of food consumption. Other researchers have demonstrated that when people are offered a choice about what food they will eat, they will choose MSG-containing foods. Further, the team of P.J. Rogers and J.E. Blundell documented that when research subjects consumed food with MSG, their desire and motivation to eat again returned more rapidly.

Scientists have known since the 1960s that MSG is a contributor to the obesity epidemic, and extensive research conducted with animals and humans clearly demonstrates a connection between MSG, obesity, and food addiction. One study randomly sampled 752 people from three rural Chinese villages. Results showed that people who consumed greater amounts of MSG were thirty percent more likely to become overweight than others whose consumption was moderate, and that those who consumed the most MSG were more than twice as likely as other study participants to become overweight. In *The Slow Poisoning of America*, scientist John Erb refers to more than five hundred studies that show a correlation between MSG and weight gain in rodents. One study showed that day-old mice and rats injected with MSG soon became overweight and developed a tendency toward diabetes. This connection between MSG and weight gain in rodents has become so commonplace that scientists refer to a generic experiment type of mouse called the "MSG-obese mouse." These mice, according to one science writer, look like inflated balloons in a parade.

A patient who struggled with binge eating for many years described how addicted she was to Chinese food. She recounted stories of having intense thoughts and cravings for specific Chinese food whenever she saw signs from the highway for Chinatown in Boston or was anywhere close to that neighborhood. She frequently drove out of her way to get Chinese food and clearly described the image of the Chinese food in her head that created hunger pangs and cravings *regardless* of when she had last eaten.

In addition to the overproduction of insulin that is triggered by MSG, another reason that MSG is linked to obesity is that it causes appetite to return more quickly and in full force, setting an addictive process in motion. This happens because MSG stimulates the pancreas to overproduce insulin. Once insulin rushes into the bloodstream, it stores excess sugar as fat and blood sugar levels drop. At this point, shortly after having eaten, the person becomes hungry, tired, and ready to eat again. MSG also blunts the effects of the hypothalamus, increasing food intake and leading to weight gain by dysregulating the body's hunger and appetite signals. These effects of MSG are all the more dangerous because they happen outside of our conscious awareness. We feel ravenous an hour after leaving a Chinese restaurant or keep returning to the pantry for more junk food without realizing we are caught up in an addictive maelstrom.

Beyond its effects on insulin, weight, and food cravings, MSG also lowers dopamine levels and increases prolactin, both of which can exacerbate depression. One study cited a forty-two percent increase in depression associated with fast food consumption. Another study found that the more fast food and processed baked goods people eat, the greater their risk of depression is.

Aside from the health consequences described above, MSG causes a host of other adverse physical ailments. In fact, soon after MSG became a popular additive in American food, American clinicians recognized a cluster of damaging effects in some people who consumed it that has now been called the *MSG complex*. MSG complex symptoms vary, but can include headaches, drowsiness, and weakness.

Symptoms of MSG Complex

- Tingling and numbness
- Burning sensation
- Facial pressure or tightness
- Chest pain or difficulty breathing
- Skin rash
- Nausea
- Rapid heartbeat
- Drowsiness
- Weakness
- Migraine headache

The food industry has responded to scientific studies highlighting the damaging effects of MSG by arguing that glutamate is a neurotransmitter found in natural foods such as tomatoes, seaweed, and milk. In fact, our first exposure to the taste of glutamate comes from breast milk. But the glutamate that exists naturally is bound in amino acid groupings rather than as free glutamate, which is the case in MSG. The free glutamic acid that comes from MSG enters the bloodstream ten times faster than natural or bound glutamate. While glutamate is normally found in minute concentrations in the brain, the free glutamic acid from MSG causes glutamate concentrations to rise and neurons to fire excessively, setting in motion an addictive cycle of exaggerated reward, withdrawal, and craving that contributes to binge eating.

Because of the scientific evidence indicating the negative health effects of MSG, the US Food and Drug Administration requires that manufacturers using MSG in their foods list it as an ingredient on their food labels. As adding MSG to ingredient lists is now widely considered controversial, manufacturers have turned their attention to other sources of free glutamic acid to avoid declaring that their products contain MSG. They now list ingredients such as yeast extract, hydrolyzed protein, calcium caseinate, sodium caseinate, textured protein, hydrolyzed corn gluten, and autolyzed yeast, substances that most consumers do not know actually contain MSG. It is important to educate yourself about food labels and understand the many different ingredients that contain MSG.

Ingredients that *always* contain MSG or processed free glutamic acid:

- Glutamic acid
- Glutamate
- Monosodium glutamate
- Monopotassium glutamate
- Calcium glutamate
- Monoammonium glutamate
- Magnesium glutamate
- Natrium glutamate
- Yeast extract
- Anything "hydrolyzed"
- Any "hydrolyzed protein"
- Calcium caseinate
- Sodium caseinate
- Yeast food, Yeast nutrient
- Autolyzed yeast
- Gelatin
- Textured protein
- Soy protein
- Soy protein concentrate
- Soy protein isolate
- Whey protein
- Whey protein concentrate
- Whey protein isolate

- Vetsin
- Ajinomoto

Ingredients that *often* contain or produce processed free glutamic acid:

- Carrageenan
- Bouillon and broth
- Stock
- Any "flavors" or "flavoring"
- Maltodextrin
- Citric acid or Citrate
- Anything "ultrapasteurized"
- Barley malt
- Pectin
- Protease
- Anything "enzyme modified"
- Anything containing "enzymes"
- Malt extract
- Soy sauce
- Soy sauce extract
- Anything "protein fortified"
- Anything "fermented"
- Seasonings

Ingredients *suspected* of containing or creating sufficient processed free glutamic acid to serve as MSG-reaction triggers in highly sensitive people:

- Corn starch
- Corn syrup
- Dextrose
- Rice syrup
- Brown rice syrup

- Milk powder
- Modified food starch
- Lipolyzed butterfat
- Reduced fat milk
- Most things low fat or no fat
- Anything vitamin enriched

MSG is everywhere, which makes it difficult to avoid unless you stay vigilant. MSG is an *excitotoxin*, meaning it "excites" cells in your body, putting them into overdrive, which ultimately leads to cell death. This cellular excitation also leads to a pattern of addiction, because after the cells have been excited by MSG, the food additive's effect upon the cells comes to an abrupt halt, triggering an increased appetite that interferes with the body's natural hunger and satiety signals.

MSG has an indirect role in food addiction and binge eating. Inspecting food labels not only for the abbreviation "MSG" but also for the plethora of code names that the food industry uses to disguise it, as well as cutting down on your consumption of fast and processed foods, will decrease your ingestion of MSG and can help address binge eating behaviors.

Summary

Monosodium glutamate, more commonly known as MSG, is a popular food additive that is treasured for its unique savory flavor and ability to enhance the overall palatability of foods. Manufacturers of packaged, frozen, and fast foods often use MSG as a quick, inexpensive way to restore the appeal that is lost during industrial processing. Yet the allure of MSG goes far beyond its taste. This coveted compound has been shown to significantly alter the biochemistry of the body and amplify food cravings, predisposing individuals to addiction. Studies have revealed that MSG stimulates appetite, suppresses satiety signals, and initiates a flush of dopamine that chemically overrides one's ability to stop eating. Once in the body, MSG acts as an excitotoxin—a chemical that aggravates cells and leaves behind a state of hormonal and metabolic turmoil. MSG has been strongly linked to chronic health problems such as obesity and diabetes, as well as a medley of acute physical complications referred to as the MSG Complex. Sensitive individuals will rapidly experience such symptoms as headaches, digestive upset, nausea, skin rash, tingling, and weakness among others.

Due to its increasingly worrisome reputation, manufacturers have started to disguise MSG under different names on food packaging. As a consumer, it is thus important to become familiar with the numerous terms used to describe MSG, and to learn how to scan food labels carefully to identify them. Avoiding MSG-containing foods can be a critical step in breaking free of food addiction and bringing appetite back into a state of balance.

Key Points

- Monosodium glutamate (MSG) is a food additive that makes food taste better, so people are inclined to eat more of the foods that contain MSG.
- MSG is an excitotoxin that sends cells into overdrive, which can damage cells and kill neurons.
- This excitotoxin effect can also trigger the addiction cycle, because when cellular activity comes to an abrupt halt, it prompts a sense of withdrawal and then a craving for more food, regardless of the amount of food consumed.
- MSG stimulates overproduction of insulin, which induces blood sugar fluctuations and increased food intake, leading to weight gain and an increased likelihood of developing diabetes.
- MSG blunts the effects of the hypothalamus, increasing food intake and leading to weight gain by dysregulating the body's hunger and appetite signals.
- Consumption of MSG decreases dopamine and increases prolactin, which is associated with depression.

- To avoid having to include MSG as an ingredient in their products, food manufacturers have devised new names for MSG, so it is important to read labels and know the various code words for MSG.

14
CONTROLLING APPETITE WITH AN UN-DIET

Dr. William Beaumont, known as the "Father of Gastric Physiology," first met patient Alexis St. Martin in 1822 when he was accidentally shot in the stomach at close range by a shotgun loaded with buckshot. Dr. Beaumont treated the wound, although he was unsuccessful in fully closing the open hole in St. Martin's stomach. Despite a poor prognosis, St. Martin survived and was subsequently hired by Dr. Beaumont as the family's handyman. In 1825, Dr. Beaumont began medical testing with St. Martin and recorded his results.

Dr. Beaumont realized the unique opportunity St. Martin presented for the real-time observation of human digestion. Most of Dr. Beaumont's experiments involved him tying a piece of food to a string and inserting it through the hole directly into St. Martin's stomach. Dr. Beaumont would inspect the food over a period of time and observe the rate of digestion of different foods. St. Martin would at times become irritable during these experiments, which led Dr. Beaumont to make an important discovery: stress can hinder digestion.

Almost two hundred years later, the medical community is still untangling the connection between stress, digestion, and the regulation of appetite. Awareness has been growing as to the importance of *how* we eat, not just *what* we eat.

James Greenblatt, MD

Mindful Eating

Mindful eating occurs when you engage and focus your full attention upon the experience of eating—the smells, tastes, thoughts, and feelings. You're conscious and aware of all aspects of the process. Many of you eat even when you're not hungry, or eat for comfort, or use food as a distraction. When you eat mindlessly, you become unaware of the dangerous effects that food can have on your emotional and physical health. By tuning all of your senses into the food you're eating, meals become more enjoyable and satisfying.

The practice of *mindfulness* starts with increasing self-awareness and living deliberately. This involves turning off the autopilot that steers us mindlessly through life and instead focusing our attentions on our thoughts, bodily sensations, and feelings. Once we are no longer "zoned out," we can begin to question knee-jerk decisions that eliminate choices. Harvard psychologist Ellen Langer calls this attitude the "power of possibility," and challenges people to become more aware of what could be rather than assuming life will go on as it always has. Langer writes that one of the most painful aspects of depression is the belief that it has lasted since time began and will be our perpetual companion. If we pay closer attention, she insists, even when we are depressed, we realize that we are not depressed every minute of every day. Recognizing that the problem is not with us constantly helps us acquire the power to manage it.

Just as the practice of mindfulness has helped people overcome depression, anxiety, stress, and chronic pain, it is also very useful in overcoming disordered eating. Relaxation exercises that focus on awareness can be transferred to eating habits and the thoughts that both prompt and maintain them. A recent review published in the journal *Eating Disorders* found that mindfulness-based eating awareness training decreased binge episodes, improved a sense of control over eating, and cultivated self-acceptance in patients with a history of disordered eating.

Two of the most common mindfulness-based therapies are *Transcendental Meditation* (TM) and *Mindfulness Based Stress Reduction* (MBSR). While MBSR emphasizes calming stress and TM cultivates transcendence of everyday problems, both utilize the discipline of meditation to support recovery from food addiction. These therapies help you to control impulsive urges and develop patience.

Science supports the benefits of meditation that individuals report anecdotally. A study of regular meditators concluded that they release sixty-five percent more dopamine into the ventral striatum than those who do not meditate. These increased levels of dopamine, sustained by meditation, reduce impulsivity and help curb food cravings.

Mindful eating is the opposite of mindless eating, during which food is consumed without awareness or enjoyment. Mindful eating involves much more than the actual process of eating; it encourages you to explore why you eat and to contemplate the roles food plays in your life that may in fact have little to do with hunger. As you eat more deliberately, you may be surprised to discover the myriad ways you rely upon food to control your moods: for instance, you drink coffee when you're tired, eat chocolate when you're sad, or raid the refrigerator when you're bored. These are knee-jerk reactions to outside stressors that can cause more problems than they solve. Mindfulness will help you uncover the automatic choices you are accustomed to making, and realize it is possible to make new and different choices.

I encourage you to un-diet, by which I mean to slow down, tune into your body's own natural signals, and eat mindfully. Mindful eating involves not only focusing deliberately on what you eat—paying attention to food textures and colors, savoring its flavors—but also on how you eat. The principles described below are elements of mindful eating that will help you transform how you eat and support a healthy relationship with food.

Eat Regular Meals

Mindful eating involves keeping the body adequately fed. This means maintaining a pattern of regular meals and snacks. Trying to manipulate what you eat by dieting, fasting, skipping meals, eliminating entire food groups, purging, or other methods will cause an effect opposite to that which you intend. Skipping meals or otherwise eating irregularly, even if only at breakfast, puts the body into a self-preservation mode that originally protected our species during famine. The body automatically slows the calorie burning rate and releases extra insulin, thereby lowering blood sugar and increasing hunger, specifically a craving for sweets.

Your mind also starts to play tricks on you when you are not getting enough food. You can find yourself constantly thinking about it; you might even dream about it. You may spend inordinate amounts of time clipping recipes, planning menus, and cooking elaborate meals for others that you plan not to touch. Isolation seems preferable, as it takes too much energy to be with others. This results in depression, anxiety, and a loss of self-esteem.

We have known for more than fifty years about some of the psychological and physical symptoms of semi-starvation. In the 1950s, researcher Ancel Keys led the Minnesota Starvation Experiment to investigate the effects of caloric restriction. The study was intended to simulate a famine and to acquire a base of scientific evidence that would guide Allied relief for famine victims in Europe and Asia at the end of World War II. Keys recruited thirty-six physically and psychologically healthy young men to participate in a year-long experiment. For the first three months, the men ate normally. During the next six months, they received only about half the original amount of food. Then, for the final three months, they were allowed to eat as much as they wanted. During the six-month period of semi-starvation, the men became obsessed with food, talking and daydreaming about it constantly. They spent much of each day planning how they would use that day's allotment of food, reading recipes and planning elaborate meals. As time passed, the men became more and more depressed, anxious, irritable, and angry. When they could finally eat again without restriction, the men "ate more or less continuously," and remained hungry even after they had finished their meals. Some consumed as much as eight thousand to ten thousand calories a day and still didn't feel a sense of satiety. Although most of the men returned to normal within five months of study completion, some continued their "extreme overconsumption." Clearly, over-restriction of food wrought havoc with appetite.

As food deprivation creates multiple psychological and physiological disturbances, try not to go for more than about three hours without a meal or snack. As your eating schedule normalizes, the body's signals of hunger and satiety should normalize as well. Eating meals at irregular times and skipping meals throws the digestive system out of sync. Eating meals on a reasonable schedule, on the other hand, regulates metabolism and maintains the pace of the digestive process. Also keep in mind that the chemical reactions in the body that form the basis of metabolism are at peak function during the day.

Slow Down

In addition to a regular mealtime schedule, mindful eating involves the establishment of a relaxing eating context. Sit down and try to keep mealtime free of distractions. If you focus on balancing your checkbook or planning your strategy for an upcoming difficult meeting, you will be unable to enjoy what you're eating or to remain attuned to your body's cues when you have had enough.

In his book *The Slow Down Diet*, author Marc David highlights the role of stress in weight gain. Our *autonomic nervous system* (ANS) regulates the functions of our internal organs as well as our *peripheral nervous system* that controls our fight-or-flight response. The ANS is divided into the *sympathetic nervous system* and the *parasympathetic nervous system*. When we are stressed, our body's sympathetic nervous system mediates the hormonal and neuronal stress response, activating our fight-or-flight response involuntarily. When we are relaxed, the parasympathetic nervous system does the opposite. Our heart rate slows down and our blood pressure decreases. The parasympathetic branch relaxes the body and activates digestion, while the sympathetic branch activates stress and suppresses digestion. When one branch is activated, the other is not. In other words, the same part of the brain that switches *on* stress switches *off* digestion. A person under stress is not physiologically able to digest and assimilate food! Remember Dr. Beaumont's studies in 1825: as the stress response increases, digestion shuts down. When the relaxation response is dominant, digestion moves in full force.

Stress contributes to a legion of problems related to digestion and disordered eating, including:

- Decreased nutrient absorption
- Increased salt retention
- Increased cortisol, linked to weight gain and abdominal obesity
- Decreased thyroid activity, which slows down metabolism.

A stressed eater has a dominant sympathetic system, which leads to digestive shutdown. A relaxed, mindful eater experiences parasympathetic dominance, and his digestive system operates at an optimal level. Restrictive eating in combination with stress sets the stage for binge eating disorder.

Many of the patients that I treat for binge eating have lived with significant stressors for years before they finally seek treatment. It appears that trauma and chronic stress disrupts the digestive system and shifts the stress response to the always "on" position. Many of you have attempted to eat well, exercise, and relax, but without repairing and optimizing nutritional deficiencies and digestive dysfunctions from the past, recovery is slow and relapse common.

The Pleasure of Eating

Relaxed meals revive pleasure in eating. Many people who have grappled with disordered eating have lost a sense of association between eating and pleasure altogether. If we deny ourselves the pleasure of food by restricting, the body responds by *demanding*, with increasing vehemence, pleasure and satisfaction. If, on the other hand, we allow ourselves to enjoy eating, the endorphins released by eating produce pleasure and stimulate the mobilization of fat. Moreover, the greater the endorphin release in the digestive tract, the more blood and oxygen will be delivered there. All this leads to more efficiency in digestion, assimilation and, ultimately, calorie burning.

Conversely, the production of excess cortisol that is triggered by stress or anxiety desensitizes us to pleasure. We tend to overeat most when we are stressed, anxious, or unaware. And – ironically – any anxiety or stress that we experience about eating makes us eat more in an effort to achieve satisfaction.

In trying to relax and enjoy mealtimes, we have a lot to learn from the French. Mireille Guilian, in her book *French Women Don't Get Fat*, reveals the secret of French women: they make a ritual out of eating every meal. French women tend to emphasize flavor and food variety over quantity, and it is not unusual for them to linger over lunch or dinner for two or three hours.

Many scientists have tried to explain "the French paradox": although Europeans eat more fat than Americans, they do not display the same increases in cholesterol and heart disease. Some think the lower rate of heart disease among the French is attributable to the red wine they drink, and some have isolated it as an effect of polyphenols, the active chemical components of red wine. Many now believe the difference is attributable to the fact that the French take their time when eating and place a high value upon the enjoyment of high-quality foods.

Choosing foods that are high in quality is an excellent nutritional strategy because high quality generally means greater nutritional value. When you eat processed foods devoid of nutrients, the brain registers a nutrient deficit and signals us to eat more. No matter what food you eat, choose foods that are fresh, locally produced, and nutrient dense.

Looking at how we eat leads to self-awareness. Mindless eating is often only a part of mindless living. A hurried and stressful relationship with food often reflects a sense of disconnection from life itself. Acknowledging this sense of being out of touch can lead the way to recognizing negative thinking patterns or to tapping into your hunger for deeper spiritual nourishment. Each of us has a story that can illuminate our relationship with food, one which may have operated in our lives for a long time. In addition, we all hold the power to rewrite our stories and to trade old, ineffective patterns for healthier, happier ones.

The scientific community has finally proven that dieting is *not* a healthy way to live. Meticulous calorie counting, portion weighing, and rigid adherence to rules take the pleasure out of eating. Dieting leads to a preoccupation with a body image. Chronic deprivation from restrictive eating, in tandem with binge eating, severely disrupts metabolism in addition to undermining the potential for happiness and psychological health.

You can learn to control your appetite and rewrite your life script free of diets. You can transform the functioning of your digestive system, limit foods that contribute to disordered eating, and eat mindfully. Unlike dieting, this – the New Hope model – is a pattern that you can sustain for a lifetime.

Summary

Despite marketing and media hype, diets and diet products are ineffective and not sustainable in the long-term. Trying to control the diet with a regimented food plan, counting calories, under-eating, or skipping meals only increases biochemical cravings and obsessive thoughts around food. A more effective way to normalize eating patterns and achieve a healthy weight is to work with the body to optimize nutritional status, stabilize blood sugar levels, and learn to trust appetite once again.

Adopting mindful practices around meal and snack times can ease the stress and emotional strain that often surrounds food. It is helpful to work towards consuming regular meals and snacks, making mealtimes as relaxing as possible, rediscovering the pleasures of eating, and putting food in perspective. When you limit foods that contribute to disordered eating habits, you're able to improve digestive function and rediscover the joy of eating. Your appetite will settle, and you will restore a positive relationship with food.

Key Points

- Diets don't work.
- Dieting disrupts natural hunger cues and destabilizes appetite in a way that causes significant stress and emotional strain.
- Slow down while you eat. When your heart rate and blood pressure decrease, digestion can operate at an optimal level. When you are stressed, you are physiologically unable to digest properly.
- Instead of following a strict food plan for weight loss, it is more helpful to stabilize appetite by putting an end to counting calories, skipping meals, and intentionally undereating.
- Optimize the way you eat mindfully. Consume regular meals and snacks, make mealtimes as relaxing as possible, rediscover the pleasure of eating, and put eating in perspective.

15
REDISCOVERING HOPE THROUGH THERAPY

This book has focused on the biochemical causes of disordered eating and ways to restore a healthy relationship with food through diet, amino acid supplements, and medications as needed. These interventions form the basis of the molecular magic that can help you step off the roller coaster and enjoy healthy eating.

But the road back to well-being often involves more than establishing healthy patterns of eating. It also involves building on inner strengths and exploring the potential of meaningful connections with the outside world. It is just as important to nurture the mind as it is to nourish the brain. Psychotherapy and interpersonal connections are additional components of the New Hope model for reclaiming a healthy appetite.

It is important to examine disordered eating within the context of all aspects of your life. What elicits and sustains your eating patterns and influences your prospects of recovery depends upon an interaction of psychological, social, and cultural factors in combination with your genetics and biochemistry. Your biochemistry is not an entity separate from your thinking style, personal values, and life experience.

Just as an individual's personality traits, beliefs, and expectations can influence the development of an addiction to food, they can also heal. Western medicine considers the patient as a passive entity to be made compliant. The reality is more complicated, and you must take an active role in examining the assumptions, beliefs, and behaviors that keep you mired in an addictive relationship with food.

If you are struggling with weight and binge eating, you likely are hostage to negative thoughts and feelings. You may think obsessively, pursuing a long chain of pervasive, negative contemplations. You may regret the past, find the present empty, and lack hope for the future. Dr. Daniel Amen characterizes this pattern of thinking as being confined by *automatic negative thoughts*, or ANTs. Thoughts are 'automatic' because you make assumptions about yourself without shining an objective, skeptical light on them. For instance, giving in once to the urge to binge confirms your view of yourself as a total failure. If you feel stuck on a roller-coaster ride, these assumptions invariably limit progress and prevent recovery. The New Hope plan will help you move beyond negative thinking toward a future of regular eating and balance.

Psychotherapy is important in the process of becoming more aware of the complicated emotions surrounding food and appetite. Cognitive-behavioral therapy (CBT) is the most well-proven form of therapy for binge eating disorder.

Cognitive-Behavioral Therapy

While many different types of therapy are available, a preponderance of research points to *cognitive-behavioral therapy* (CBT) as being the most effective for the treatment of disordered eating. CBT involves your active participation in understanding the behavioral and emotional components embedded in chronic disordered eating patterns. Rather than exploring the past or searching for root causes of problem behaviors in early family dynamics, CBT addresses issues in your present life. The therapist helps you explore self-perpetuating beliefs and examine the emotions and thought processes that may in fact be trapping you in cyclic patterns of destructive behavior.

CBT maintains that thoughts (or cognitions), feelings, and behaviors operate in a feedback loop. If the perception that you are a bad person looms continuously in your mind, you will feel sadness and a sense of shame. You may distract yourself from these painful feelings through bingeing, purging, or other disordered eating behaviors. Similarly, how you act affects your thoughts and feelings. For example, if you eat a slice of cake and believe that this action confirms your lack of willpower, you will feel guilty and worthless. As you tend towards all-or-nothing thinking, you are increasingly likely to decide you might as well eat the rest of the cake.

CBT therapists can help you interrupt this feedback loop by deconstructing your thoughts and questioning the logic underlying these negative judgments. Once corrosive and critical self-assessments are replaced by more hopeful and forgiving—as well as realistic—ones, mood lifts. As you become conscious of the thoughts that were once automatic, you can learn to challenge these assumptions on your own and help yourself heal. Unsurprisingly, CBT has been shown to be just as effective in treating depression as antidepressant medication, and even better than antidepressants at preventing relapse.

CBT does not stop with changing patterns of thinking. It helps you to monitor your eating behaviors, and to develop strategies and alternatives for behaviors that keep old patterns in play. For example, if you tend to plan binges when you have the house to yourself, you may decide to explain this pattern to your partner. Your partner can then help you avoid having a stretch of time alone in the house. Meanwhile, you'll explore other alternatives to cope with the negative thoughts and feelings that fuel the urge to binge. By paying close attention to your patterns of eating, you may realize that the fast-food restaurant you pass on the way to work is too seductive a temptation for the time being. Deciding to take a different route is a way to adjust your behavior while you work on understanding and changing the way you feel. When you are successful at avoiding behaviors that perpetuate the cycle, you feel better about yourself.

CBT is the treatment of choice for patients with disordered eating. This is partly because the emotional context of disordered eating is based on a distorted core belief: an overvaluation of shape and weight. Eating disorders are sustained by unforgiving dietary restriction and extreme methods of weight control, which together intensify the need to binge.

Disordered eating is, as viewed through the CBT lens, akin to a house of cards. If you remove certain key cards that form the scaffolding, then you bring down the entire house.

A recent study reinforces results from earlier investigations that suggest CBT is the best treatment for binge eating and disordered eating behaviors. Conducted by Danish researchers, this study compared the effectiveness of CBT with psychoanalytic psychotherapy in treating bulimia nervosa. Half the patients were treated with psychoanalytic psychotherapy, which involved regular meetings with a psychoanalyst to uncover the deep feelings and early conflicts that may have led to bulimia. The therapists who met with the other half of the patients used CBT to target symptoms and show patients how to challenge the beliefs that maintain them. The therapists then helped the patients adopt more flexible, realistic guidelines and anticipate binges in order to mitigate their symptom severity.

The researchers conducting the study reached a conclusion that surprised them. Even though the patients who received psychoanalytic psychotherapy met much more frequently with the therapist, the patients who received CBT realized significantly better outcomes. Five months after the start of the trial, six percent of patients undergoing psychoanalytic psychotherapy stopped bingeing and purging; forty-two percent of those receiving CBT had stopped bingeing and purging in the same timeframe. After two years, fifteen percent of those treated with psychoanalytic psychotherapy were free of bingeing and purging behaviors, as compared with a total of forty-four percent of those receiving CBT.

These study results are all the more surprising—and a credit to the investigators' clear-eyed, unbiased research—because the lead investigators are, themselves, psychoanalysts.

One other study about CBT deserves mention. In the next chapter of this book, you will read about other lifestyle interventions that are important to the New Hope model. One of these is exercise. A study conducted in Australia attests to the efficacy of adding exercise to CBT in patients with binge eating disorder. The study used exercise as an adjunct to CBT in one of the treatment groups and found that the patients who exercised also binged less than those who received CBT alone. In addition, those who exercised lost weight throughout the study, while those who did not exercise stayed the same or gained some weight despite a decrease in binges. The researchers speculate that adding an exercise activity to treatment with CBT may benefit binge eaters both *physiologically*—their bodies burn calories at a higher rate—and *psychologically*—they enjoy the pleasure of recreation and enhanced self-esteem. In other words, adding exercise to a treatment program for disordered eating can support the hopeful reframing of thinking and experience that is the goal of CBT.

Motivational Interviewing

Motivational interviewing, a client-centered counseling approach pioneered by clinical psychologists William R. Miller and Stephen Rollnick, works by eliciting a patient's intrinsic motivation to change a behavior. The approach is neither judgmental nor confrontational; instead, it focuses on helping people resolve their ambivalence towards problematic behaviors and then proactively change the behaviors. Motivational interviewing was first used and found to be successful in treating problem drinkers.

Recently, motivational interviewing has been shown to be effective in treating binge eating. One study involving ninety patients with either non-purging bulimia nervosa or binge eating disorder compared the efficacy of self-help to an intervention which combined self-help with motivational interviewing. A significantly greater number of the participants who received the combined intervention binged less and felt better about themselves than did those who had just received self-help. Another randomized controlled trial compared the benefits of motivational interviewing and self-help with an educational intervention plus self-help in patients with binge eating disorder and bulimia. This study also documented greater improvement amongst patients who had received motivational interviewing.

These studies suggest that motivational interviewing holds promise for the treatment of binge eating. Motivational interviewing appears to help people accelerate their readiness to stop bingeing, and to improve their sense of self-control. In addition, the therapy is both brief and inexpensive.

Family-Based Therapy

While CBT seems to be the most promising form of psychotherapy for a majority of people with eating disorders, it is not always the best treatment for adolescents. CBT encourages individuals to take responsibility for behaviors. Most adolescents are not yet responsible for organizing meals at home. Moreover, adolescents generally still live at home with their families and under the authority of their parents.

Family therapy can help detoxify the emotional context that may develop around an adolescent's eating behaviors. Parents often feel tremendous guilt in relation to their child's disordered eating, or take their child's lapses from normal eating personally. A family therapist can help parents work through such reactions and mobilize their own strengths as the best allies in their child's efforts to regain a healthy appetite.

As with other types of therapy, different models of family therapy are available. One type that has been successful with disordered eating, especially anorexia nervosa, is the *Maudsley model*. Named for the London hospital where it was developed more than twenty years ago, the Maudsley model involves the entire family—patient, parents, and siblings. During sessions, the family is asked to join together to confront and ultimately solve the problem of disordered eating.

Treatment occurs in three phases. The first phase is characterized by intensive parental involvement. The parents are taught to present a unified front to the adolescent. If the patient's mother has kept in confidence her daughter's tendency to vomit after meals, she is guided to acknowledge the importance of sharing this secret with the rest of the family. Facing a problem honestly and directly as a family team builds the likelihood of success. The parents prepare all meals for their adolescent child and join her when she eats during this initial phase. In the next phase, the patient is gradually allowed to regain control of her eating habits. The final phase focuses on helping the adolescent establish autonomy, develop relationships that have normal boundaries, and return to typical teen activities.

Family-based therapy has been successful in adolescents with bulimia in addition to those with anorexia. Several studies comparing the relative benefits of family-based therapy and supportive individual psychotherapy have reported greater benefits from family-based therapy. One British study compared the Maudsley method to individual supportive therapy in fifty-seven patients with anorexia nervosa and twenty-three with bulimia nervosa. A higher percentage of adolescents who underwent family-based therapy were free of eating disorder symptoms five years after treatment than those who participated in individual supportive therapy. In a randomized controlled comparison of family-based therapy and supportive psychotherapy for adolescents with bulimia, thirty-nine percent of those undergoing family-based therapy and eighteen percent of those in individual therapy had stopped bingeing and purging when the study ended. Although not all of these adolescents were abstinent a year later, a higher percentage of those who had undergone family therapy treatment remained abstinent. These researchers are still exploring ways to increase the recovery success rates from disordered eating amongst adolescents, and they believe family involvement is key. Because of the proven effectiveness of cognitive-behavioral therapy, *integrative CBT with family-based treatment* can be the most beneficial interventions for adolescents and families.

Group Therapy

Group therapy presents another opportunity for active participation in your recovery from disordered eating. For many, involvement in a supportive group can constitute the most important component of therapy. In a study conducted in Israel, researcher Arthur Trokzky divided adolescent female participants with disordered eating into two intervention groups. The first was treated with group therapy in sessions that were co-led by the researcher and a person who had suffered from food addiction. The other participants were seen in individual therapy. Dr. Trotzky found a significantly higher recovery rate among those who were treated in the group setting. Recovery, measured by weight loss and a cessation of purging behaviors, was documented in sixty-two percent of those treated in group therapy, versus thirty-three percent of those treated in individual sessions.

The federal government organization designated to treat substance abuse, the Substance Abuse and Mental Health Services Administration, or SAMHSA, now recommends group therapy as the preferred method for treating substance abuse. Groups have several fundamental advantages for this kind of treatment, as there are intrinsic rewards to participating in group programs. First, they offer positive support from peers as well as peer pressure to abstain from addictive behaviors. Members can also challenge each other in a caring way about self-destructive tendencies, irrational thinking, and inconsistencies in thought and behavior. This type of interaction helps participants learn to express anger, disappointment, and other negative feelings in a constructive manner—a very important life skill. Many people who struggle with disordered eating have trouble expressing negative feelings; they tend to "swallow" their hurt or rage rather than expressing it directly. Learning to recognize and voice negative feelings in a safe and supportive setting can enhance opportunities to actively and honestly participate in all aspects of recovery.

Groups also reduce isolation, an important benefit for people who have shied away from others out of shame. Groups enable participants to witness the struggles and triumphs of other members, and to see firsthand that recovery is possible. In addition, they show how others cope with stresses. Members often coach people new to recovery as they take on tasks that may provoke anxiety. Groups can offer family-like experiences, enabling participants to learn social skills in a protected environment. Perhaps most importantly, groups can provide the hope and inspiration that is needed to get off the roller coaster of disordered eating.

Group therapy for food addiction is not the same as a support group such as Overeaters Anonymous (OA). Support groups have their own treatment niche as well. OA is a twelve-step program similar to Alcoholics Anonymous (AA), which has helped hundreds of thousands of people recover from alcoholism. OA and other twelve-step programs are run by members of the group itself rather than by a mental health professional. Although the meeting discussions are not likely to be as probing as those in group therapy, OA can be a powerful adjunct to treating food addiction. OA meetings are free, and are available in major cities every day of the week and sometimes at different times of day. They can provide immediate help in controlling food urges when a group therapy appointment may still be days away. And self-led support groups provide some of the same benefits as group therapy in that members share a common problem in a safe environment. Please see the Resources section for information on other support groups for recovery from food addiction and binge eating.

Hypnotherapy

Another treatment for disordered eating is *hypnotherapy*. Hypnosis has been used in therapy since the time of Sigmund Freud at the end of the nineteenth century. Freud used hypnosis to unlock the unconscious mind, hoping to bring to light motivations behind distressing behavior that were inaccessible through traditional conversation. While its use in magic performances and county fairs has tarnished its image, research shows that hypnosis is not just a gimmick or an entertaining stage show. Hypnotherapy does not involve the stereotypical swinging of a pocket watch in front of someone's face, lulling him or her into a state of mind beyond conscious control. Rather, hypnotherapy involves using relaxation techniques such as visualization to put a person into a state of highly focused attention undisturbed by outside distractions. This state is reflected in brain imaging studies that show that hypnosis increases theta waves, which are associated with dreaming and meditation. In this state, you are suggestible to comments made by the practitioner. The practitioner does not wield control over your thoughts or actions; instead, you are just less likely to consider alternatives to the suggestions the practitioner puts forth. You ultimately determine how you will respond to the practitioner, which means that you are in control. By hearing suggestions in this altered state, you are not mired in the typical thought patterns that brought you to therapy in the first place.

Hypnosis has been effective in helping people stop smoking. Smokers who had tried to quit multiple times were put into a relaxed and receptive state of hypnosis and therapists then made suggestions about smoking: "Cigarettes are harmful and cause uncomfortable symptoms," and "You can cope with the withdrawal symptoms." The veteran smokers were more likely to quit smoking using this method than using other treatments.

Hypnosis has also been used effectively in other contexts in medicine and mental health. After World War II, hypnosis helped reduce traumatic stress reactions in returning soldiers. Hypnosis has also been effective for anesthesia during surgery and in cases of pain from dental work, amputation, burn injuries, spinal cord injuries, lupus, and headaches. One study used hypnosis to help children undergoing a painful and distressing radiologic treatment. The researchers found that the procedure was not only less traumatic for the children, but the procedure was less difficult and time-consuming for the medical staff to perform because hypnosis lowered their patients' anxiety levels. Hypnosis has also been used to treat other forms of anxiety, depression, PTSD, and eating disorders.

Several studies have reached encouraging conclusions about the utility of hypnotherapy for disordered appetite. In a study of obesity and hypnosis, researchers noted that hypnosis improved problem solving, body image, self-esteem, motivation, and stress associated with dieting, control, and eating habits. Another study assessed the benefits of hypnosis in conjunction with CBT and found that the patient group also treated with hypnotherapy achieved better impulse control than those treated with CBT alone. In all of these studies, what researchers found most promising about hypnosis is that people can learn to use the skills of self-hypnosis for prolonged periods. This increases your sense of hope and self-efficacy in tackling problems with binge eating and food addiction.

Emotional Freedom Technique

Emotional Freedom Technique (EFT) can also benefit those dealing with binge eating disorder or other appetite problems. EFT is a type of energy psychology developed by Gary Craig in the 1990s which, like acupuncture, perceives the human body as a system of electricity and energy fields. Blockages in the natural flow of energy result in physical and emotional problems. To eliminate these problems, the blockages must be cleared. Unlike acupuncture, EFT does not use needles; instead, it involves tapping on acupressure points on the body in order to release trapped energy. It also incorporates elements of cognitive therapy in that the clinician may talk about the problem while tapping, exposing the patient to uncomfortable feelings, and then assist the patient in reframing the problem. For example, someone with binge eating disorder may feel helpless to stop eating once a meal has begun. Using EFT, you would tap on specific acupressure points while talking about your sense of helplessness and focusing on the negative feelings associated with eating a meal in this emotional state. After tapping on the negative emotions, you then focus on accepting these feelings. This acceptance leads you to an emotional crossroads: you may choose to no longer feel helpless whenever you eat.

Research on EFT is still relatively new and results are mixed. Studies using functional MRIs have shown that tapping on acupressure points releases neurotransmitters in the limbic system of the brain, which induces relaxation and calms the fight-or-flight response. Even though the results of research studies are still inconclusive, you may find EFT helpful. I believe it is particularly applicable for people struggling with food and eating problems because eating or bingeing is often a coping mechanism to deal with painful feelings. By using EFT, you can "tap on" difficult emotions and experiences, and actually alter the brain's response to these issues. Finding your problems more bearable, you may find you need to rely less upon food to distract yourself from them.

James Greenblatt, MD

Many Therapeutic Options Are Available

There are many options for therapy available to help you control binge eating and an appetite gone wild. Although CBT has been shown to be the most helpful for binge eating among large study groups, this does not mean it is necessarily the best for every individual. Longer-term *psychodynamic therapy* can also help patients with disordered eating, particularly if you are trying to address not only one problem behavior but a difficult past that shadows other aspects of your life. *Psychoanalytic therapy* delves deeper into the roots of your emotions, often exploring unconscious motives and defenses, thereby helping you move beyond self-destructive behaviors over time.

Although there are different schools of therapy, research suggests that a patient's trusting relationship with a therapist is more important than the therapist's conceptual methodology. If interpersonal difficulties have been a factor in disordered eating, the opportunity to work some of these out with a person who does not react in the predictable (and sometimes dysfunctional) ways of family members can help you move beyond these problems. You become a partner with your therapist in regaining health, control, and hope.

The opportunity to tell your story is important in and of itself, as our view of ourselves is shaped by the stories we tell. Current research shows that the way you describe an occurrence determines the choices or lack of choices you see. The opportunity to rework your personal story with a therapist can help you envision a more hopeful future.

Family and friends can be therapeutic. Connections with others will help you emerge from the isolation and shame of weight and chaotic eating patterns. I have observed that some patients—often very successful professionals—come to my office alone and are secretive about their struggles with food. Others come with a spouse or other family member. Those accompanied by supportive family members tend to continue their treatment and are more likely to achieve relief from the symptoms of disordered eating than those who keep their struggles a secret.

Whether you choose CBT, family-based therapy, group therapy, or some other combination, I believe that involvement in therapy provides an important answer to binge eating. Although your struggles with appetite have biological components, the body is not an entity separate from the mind. Integrative medicine maintains that the problems that affect our bodies are interwoven in complex ways with our thoughts, feelings, and behaviors. Understanding the complex connections that reinforce disordered eating is a step toward freedom from them. No longer confined by corrosive thinking, your vista will expand. What you will see is New Hope.

Summary

Although food addictions are strongly influenced by genetic features and individual biochemistry, disordered eating evolves from the dynamic interplay of both physical *and* psychological factors. Recovering from disordered eating involves more than healing the body; it requires cultivating inner strengths, developing social connections, and rebuilding positive associations within the mind. Psychotherapy can be very helpful in addressing the complex array of experiences that influence relationships with food. Therapy with an experienced clinician will provide you with a framework for processing the complex thoughts and emotions involved in disordered eating in a way that is safe and constructive. Group therapy and support groups can also be helpful for breaking the patterns of isolation and shame surrounding food addiction and can offer an understanding community in which to actively engage.

Of the many styles of psychotherapy offered today, Cognitive Behavior Therapy, or CBT, has proven to be the most helpful for people struggling with appetite disorders. The CBT approach aims to shift distorted eating behaviors by first reframing the negative thoughts and feelings that drive them. Family-based therapy is promising in adolescents, and some people find group therapy especially helpful. Preliminary research also suggests that energy-based techniques such as hypnotherapy and Emotional Freedom Technique (EFT) can also have powerful effects on improving body image, building motivation, enhancing self-esteem, and lowering stress in participants grappling with appetite control.

Establishing a safe, trusting relationship with a therapist, regardless of his or her particular style, technique, or discipline, is a very important step in recovering from disordered eating. Not only will therapy provide tools for rebuilding a positive relationship with food—it will help you to restore a meaningful, healthy connection with yourself.

Key Points

- The development of food addiction is influenced by more than biochemical and genetic attributes alone; psychological, social, and environmental factors also play a role.
- Psychotherapy provides a safe and healthy framework for exploring the complex experiences, thoughts, and emotions underlying distorted relationships with food.
- Cognitive behavioral therapy (CBT) is a treatment that helps change thought and belief patterns which can, in turn, change behaviors around food.
- Family-based therapy appears to be the most effective treatment for adolescents with disordered eating.
- Group therapy and support groups provide a space for individuals with similar struggles to discuss, problem-solve, and build relationships in a structured way. Such collaborative environments have proven very helpful in decreasing the shame and loneliness often associated with appetite problems.
- Although frequently mocked in the media, hypnotherapy is a powerful clinical tool that uses relaxation techniques such as visualization to break the cycle of addictive eating.

16
MASTERING THE BALANCE OF MOVEMENT AND SLEEP

Another lifestyle intervention that provides an answer to binge eating is mastering the balance of movement and rest. These are the yin and yang of health. Exercise is critical for all of us, especially for those who wish to reclaim a healthy relationship with food. Moderate aerobic exercise alters hormone levels in ways that curb appetite. In addition, exercise is a wonderful stress reliever. For these reasons, exercise allows you to tap into your body's natural reward system and take back control of your eating.

Sleep is as important as exercise in restoring a healthy appetite. Getting enough sleep helps regulate appetite by fostering the production of leptin, which signals the brain when the body has had enough food. Conversely, sleep deprivation contributes to both cravings for junk food and storage of fat in cells throughout the body. Making sure you get enough exercise and enough sleep is fundamental for getting off the roller coaster of disordered eating.

Exercise

Scientists have long known that increasingly sedentary lifestyles exacerbate many health problems, particularly disordered eating and weight gain. Healthcare professionals are beginning to pay more attention to the need to incorporate exercise into medical care for their patients. For instance, the Institute of Lifestyle Medicine currently offers courses through Harvard Medical School's Continuing Medical Education Program to teach physicians and other healthcare professionals how to make exercise a component of a patient's prescription.

This doesn't mean turning patients into exercise fanatics or getting them to run marathons or participate in triathlons. Instead, these medical professionals learn strategies and techniques to help patients incorporate exercise into lifestyle. Exercise is a safe and effective strategy for you in combination with supplements, medications, and therapy.

Many of you, however, must overcome significant barriers to exercise. Even though you know exercise is good for you, summoning the motivation and energy to actually do it is another story. Knowing what to do is often easier than doing what you know. A major obstacle is lack of energy. Fatigue is common among people with food and appetite problems, and for a number of reasons. First, depression is the most common mental illness associated with eating disorders and, along with low mood and various other symptoms, often manifests in somatic (bodily) symptoms such as fatigue. Whereas exercise can reduce symptoms of depression, somatic symptoms of depression can prevent you from exercising. Therefore, one of the most important things you can do to help lift a depressed mood can be one of the hardest things to do... simply because you are depressed!

Researchers exploring the underlying causes of fatigue associated with depression have found an interesting link with *mitochondria*, the energy-producing factories of every cell in the body. Mitochondria are tiny structures within cells that that generate *adenosine triphosphate* (ATP), the fuel that keeps cells running. Damage to the mitochondria means less energy is made available to cells which, consequently, will function less efficiently. Less mitochondrial energy in the brain and muscles affects the entire body. In 2008, a team of researchers from Sweden and the United States studied a possible link between mitochondrial energy and depression. They compared mitochondrial function in the muscle tissue of ten healthy people with the muscle tissue of twenty-one patients suffering from major depressive disorder who reported somatic complaints such as fatigue. The researchers concluded that mitochondrial activity was weakened in patients who experienced fatigue and depression. This research suggests a link between cellular energy levels and mood disorders.

Moreover, weight gain causes levels of mitochondria to decrease, meaning that even less energy is made available in the form of ATP. Lower ATP levels in the tissues of overweight individuals are directly correlated with fatigue and a decreased motivation to exercise. Furthermore, as ATP levels decrease, the natural response is to eat more, particularly sugar, sparking a cycle of weight gain. Cellular energy depletion leads us to consume sugar-laden foods to get a compensatory energy boost. The weight gain that occurs as a result of this process is directly linked to inefficient ATP synthesis and decreased mitochondrial production.

Fortunately, exercise can counteract these negative effects of weight gain. By increasing the number of mitochondria in the body, exercise stimulates the production of more ATP, creating more cellular energy. With more energy available, fatigue decreases and cravings for sugar diminish. Exercise can give you back the energy you need to recover from chronic patterns of disordered eating.

Exercise not only increases energy but also improves mood. Because mood and overall mental health can drive disordered eating, understanding the relationship between mood and exercise is important. Physical exercise steps up production of the neurotransmitter serotonin, which regulates emotion. When serotonin receptors are full, we feel calm and centered. When serotonin is depleted, the same neuron that initially released the chemical will soak it back up again. This prevents the serotonin from filling the nerve receptors on the next neuron. To avoid this depletion, serotonin production needs to continue so the neurons will not take the serotonin back up. This is exactly how the antidepressants known as SSRIs—selective serotonin reuptake inhibitors—work. Exercise increases serotonin production, and the effects last even after a workout session is over.

Exercise also stimulates the growth of neurons and their dendrites (*dendrites* are the tapering, branch-like extensions of neurons responsible for picking up information from neighboring neurons and transmitting the information to the neuron's *soma*, or body). Stress and anxiety, two of the most powerful factors influencing disordered eating, cause dendrites in the brain to retract, and limit the capacity of neuronal circuits to relay signals to each other. Exercise has been shown to repair this.

Physical activity has a beneficial effect on the brain's dopamine system as well. Exercise increases levels of dopamine and the number of dopamine receptors in the brain. When stressed, we search for ways to soothe ourselves and, with food cues continually invading our lives, many of us habitually reach for food. Dopamine helps to quell these cravings.

Research shows that exercise can reduce the urge to use food as a tool to cope with anxiety, stress, and depression. In one study examining the relationship between anxiety, exercise, and binge eating, researchers found that subjects who engaged in moderate exercise experienced less anxiety and indulged in fewer episodes of binge eating. Interestingly, subjects who engaged in vigorous physical exercise showed greater levels of anxiety and binge eating, demonstrating the critical importance of moderation. A number of other studies have shown that regular exercise reduces symptoms of anxiety and depressive disorders and is even associated with a lower likelihood of developing these disorders. Yoga has been shown to be particularly effective for the reduction of anxiety. A study of musicians suffering from tension, anger, and depression found that those who practiced yoga experienced a significant decrease in these negative symptoms. In another study assessing the relationship between exercise and depression over a ten-year period, it was determined that those who exercised more showed decreased symptoms of depression. The authoring researchers concluded that physical exercise counteracted the effects of negative life events and environmental stress.

So how does exercise help with hunger management? First, moderate-intensity exercise decreases hunger both during exercise and immediately afterwards. Exercise also helps shift the body's balance of peptides and hormone levels that help control appetite. Moderate exercise has been shown to lower the hunger-inducing hormone ghrelin, while increasing levels of the hormone PYY as well as GLP-1 and other polypeptides that quiet hunger. Studies have documented a decrease in ghrelin post-workout, indicating that exercise reduces hunger levels.

Research clearly establishes the importance of exercise as a component of any treatment plan for food or appetite problems. One study directly demonstrates the helpful effects of exercise in treating binge eating disorder. In a randomized trial in which half of the participants received a combination of therapy along with an exercise intervention, a total of 81.4% whose treatment included the exercise intervention stopped bingeing by the end of the study. Those who had therapy alone were not able to remain abstinent from bingeing. The authors determined that the participants were able to resist cravings because exercise stimulated highs similar to those induced by foods that characteristically triggered their binges.

Another study assessed the relative benefits of therapy, nutritional counseling, and exercise in treating bulimia nervosa. Cognitive behavioral therapy, or CBT, which we discussed in Chapter 15, is often considered the first-choice therapy for helping people address disordered eating. In this study, participants were randomly assigned to one of three treatment groups: one group received nutritional counseling, one group participated in CBT, and the third group engaged in a moderate exercise program. The fundamental concept behind the exercise program was fitness for life. Including both aerobic and nonaerobic activities, the program intended to promote physical fitness, reduce the sense of fatness and bloating resulting from being overweight, enhance body image, and prevent bingeing and purging. Participants in the exercise group enjoyed the best results. Those who received nutritional counseling alone experienced less improvement than those who had CBT, and CBT had a less positive effect than exercise. Moreover, when the positive effects of both CBT and exercise were measured after study completion, participants in the exercise group continued to enjoy a reduction in symptoms of disordered eating whilst the positive effects from CBT diminished over time.

The reduction in binge eating correlated with exercise may be due to the significant role exercise plays in interrupting addictive processes. One study conducted at Vanderbilt University assessed the impact of moderate treadmill use over a two-week period in men with a marijuana habit. On average, these men cut their smoking in half, *even when they were not asked to cut down*. After the study, those men who had found some sort of outlet in exercise reported diminished cravings for marijuana, less compulsiveness and fewer emotional ups and downs. The researchers speculated that exercise altered the reward circuits in the men's brains and replaced cannabis as a source of reward and satisfaction. The rewards of exercise became self-reinforcing.

Additional studies demonstrate the efficacy of exercise in breaking addictive patterns to other drugs. Laboratory rats exposed to exercise for six weeks became less responsive to cocaine than they had been before they began exercising. The researchers postulate that regular exercise triggered the production of enzymes responsible for creating receptors in the reward centers of the rats' brains. The creation of these receptors, they believe, resulted in the diminution of the rats' positive responses to cocaine, thereby reducing their addiction to it.

In 2007, researchers at the University of Exeter in England found that people trying to stop smoking could combat their nicotine cravings by engaging in a short, brisk walk. The investigators decided to apply this strategy to food addiction. They worked with a group of participants who were hooked on chocolate, most likely because of its mood-boosting and stress-lowering effects. Participants were required to abstain from chocolate for three days, at which point they were randomly directed either to rest or to take a walk. Afterwards, they were given a task that would be likely to trigger a chocolate craving. The participants who had walked experienced fewer cravings than the group that rested, both during the walk and afterwards. Together, the results from these studies shed light on the potential of exercise to interrupt the cycle of reward, withdrawal, and craving that is the hallmark of addiction.

For people who have been addicted to food, exercise may provide a natural substitute as it stimulates many of the same reward pathways in the brain. It also gives people healthy, long-term distractions from disordered eating. Once you begin exercising, you can tap into your body's natural reward system and take back the control that has slipped away from you. Your mood will lift, the peptides and hormones that regulate hunger and satiety will regulate, and you can improve your overall health. You are also likely to become more resilient to stress. Physiological measures such as blood pressure and heart rate and psychological measures such as anxiety and depressed mood are influenced less by stress in those who exercise regularly than in people who are inactive. Ralph Carson, in *The Brain Fix*, writes that the exercise program you choose should be 1) attainable, 2) easy to measure and 3) important to you. Once you get started, you will quickly see rewards in the form of a decrease in appetite, a general feeling of well-being, and enhanced self-esteem. This constellation of benefits is what he calls "the progressive domino effect of lifestyle change." The sooner you start a healthy exercise program, the sooner you can begin to experience these benefits!

Sleep

To bring your appetite under control, sleep is just as important as exercise. If you are surviving on less than seven or eight hours of sleep a night, you are more likely than those who get enough sleep to reach for pizza or cookies to sustain your energy during the day.

Chances are that you are among the increasing number of people not getting enough sleep. In 2001, thirty-eight percent of Americans reported getting at least eight hours of sleep per night; by 2009, that number had dipped to twenty-eight percent. The number of Americans who reported sleeping less than six hours per night rose from thirteen to twenty percent in the same time frame: one in five Americans was surviving on severely inadequate sleep.

The increase in obesity in America has occurred at the same time as the decline in average sleep duration. People who sleep less than six hours per night are more likely to gain weight, increase body fat percentage, and have a bigger waist circumference. Those who sleep less than four hours per night have a seventy-three percent chance of being considerably overweight.

If you are one of these people surviving on less than optimal sleep, sleep deprivation may be making it more difficult to control disordered eating. Sleep profoundly influences levels of hormones that are associated with appetite. Two of the most important are leptin and ghrelin. With sleep loss, levels of the appetite-suppressing hormone leptin fall, while levels of the appetite-stimulating hormone ghrelin rise.

Leptin, a hormone that is released by fat cells, signals satiety. It is produced much more sparingly in times of sleep deprivation. Moreover, leptin also plays an important role in metabolic regulation: lower levels of leptin lead to a decrease in metabolism, which, in turn, means that you have to eat less food in order to avoid gaining weight.

The second hormone, ghrelin, triggers appetite. During times of sleep deprivation, ghrelin production in the body increases, making the appetite more urgent and insistent. Considerable research reveals the interaction of sleep deprivation, ghrelin and leptin levels, and appetite. One study looked at how sleep deprivation affected ghrelin, leptin, and food consumption. Researchers in this study separated participants into two groups: one group was allowed to sleep for five hours per night for five days, while the other group slept for nine hours per night for five days. Those who were sleep-deprived had ghrelin and leptin levels that *should* have signaled satiety and the cessation of eating, yet these participants still ate more than their bodies needed, leading to weight gain over the course of the study. This finding suggests that the participants who were short on sleep ate more in order to maintain wakefulness. Moreover, they reached preferentially for carbohydrates - foods that gave them a quick burst of energy. Another study demonstrated that insufficient sleep resulted in lower levels of leptin, higher cortisol levels, and lower glucose tolerance, all of which are associated with increased food intake and abdominal fat. The researchers who conducted this study concluded that sleep deprivation contributes not only to weight gain but also to a set of risk factors associated with type 2 diabetes.

Two recent studies highlight the link between sleep deprivation and cravings for junk food. Using magnetic resonance imaging (MRI), scientists at the University of California at Berkeley scanned the brains of twenty-three healthy young adults, with the first scans taken after a normal night's sleep and repeat scans taken after a sleepless night. Second-phase scans – taken after a night of no sleep – revealed impaired activity in the participants' frontal lobes, the part of the brain that governs complex decision making. Deeper brain centers that respond to reward, however, exhibited increased activity. In addition, participants favored unhealthy junk foods while they were exhausted and sleep-deprived. The researchers concluded that high-level brain regions responsible for complex judgment are blunted by lack of sleep, whereas more primal brain structures that control motivation and desire are amplified. The combination of altered deep brain activity and impaired decision-making may help explain why people who sleep less tend to be overweight.

Another study conducted in 2012 by researchers from St. Luke's-Roosevelt Hospital Center and Columbia University revealed similar results. Researchers showed twenty-five average-weight volunteers images of healthy and unhealthy foods during MRI scans; this test was performed once after five nights of up to nine hours of sleep, and then a second time after five nights of only four hours of sleep. The reward centers of the volunteers' brains displayed significantly higher levels of activation in response to images of unhealthy food during the *second* trial - when volunteers were sleeping only four hours a night – than they did in the first trial when the volunteers were well-rested. The lead investigator concluded that the response to junk food was a neuronal pattern specific to restricted sleep. This study provides concrete evidence that we have a greater propensity to succumb to unhealthy food cravings when we are sleep-deprived. The good news is that getting a good night's sleep can quell cravings for junk food.

Sleep loss interferes with the way people process carbohydrates, and fuels stronger cravings. There is no shortage of evidence that chronic sleep deprivation is much worse than many people realize. The data make clear that getting more quality sleep can help you overcome a wide range of eating problems.

Balancing sleep with exercise, rest with movement, is key to controlling appetite. Sleep and exercise reinforce each other; when you engage in regular, moderate exercise, you are more likely to sleep well. Similarly, restful sleep helps you recover the vitality to sustain and enjoy the feeling of exercising your body. Once you make the personal investment in taking this step, you will reap dividends both day and night.

Summary

It is a well-known fact that exercise is integral to lasting strength and physical wellness. However, not until recently has the medical community fully recognized the role that physical activity plays in managing binge eating disorder and associated health complications. Engaging in a regular exercise program has been shown to boost energy levels, improve mood, and restore a metabolism that has been disrupted by food addiction. By increasing the number of mitochondria in cells, moderate exercise can also reverse the fatigue and blood sugar disarray associated with weight gain. Regular physical activity can have profound effects on the hormones and peptides involved in keeping satiety signals regular and appetite under control.

Getting an adequate amount of sleep is also crucial for maintaining proper hormone, peptide, and neurotransmitter balance. Studies have found that sleep deprivation dramatically alters brain chemistry in a way that increases the addictive potential of carbohydrates and fat-rich foods. A lack of sleep has also been correlated with unstable blood sugar levels, mood problems, and obesity, among other serious health issues. Caring for the body by engaging in a gentle exercise program and getting adequate rest can quickly reset the destructive cycle of bingeing and can help you take back your life.

Key Points

- A sedentary lifestyle contributes to many health problems, including weight gain and disordered eating.
- Health professionals are being educated on how to include exercise programs in patient care plans.

- Exercise program participation can improve energy, decrease food cravings, and help break the cycle of binge eating.
- Physical movement stimulates the production of mitochondria in the body, increasing cellular energy and reversing the fatigue associated with weight gain.
- Exercise decreases hunger and balances the peptide and hormone levels linked with appetite control.
- Gentle to moderate activity decreases anxiety and improves mood by increasing the body's feel good neurotransmitters: dopamine, serotonin, and norepinephrine.
- Getting adequate sleep is essential for maintaining proper hormone, neurotransmitter, and peptide levels.
- Sleep deprivation alters brain chemistry and triggers cravings for fat and carbohydrate-rich foods.
- A lack of sleep exacerbates high cortisol levels, low leptin stores, and unstable blood sugar, all of which are associated with obesity.
- Practicing healthy movement and getting sufficient rest will help restore biochemical balance and bring appetite back under control.

PART V.
YOUR NEW HOPE

17
SURVIVAL OF THE FATTEST

Years ago, a patient named Julie transformed my career.

Julie was a young and talented law student with a strong sense of determination. I first met her during morning rounds on the inpatient eating disorder unit. She had spent the previous two weeks at a local hospital following a suicide attempt with an overdose of multiple medications. The first few days she was in the intensive care unit, she was unconscious with a tube in her lungs to support her breathing.

Julie had overdosed in the middle of a nightly binge episode. She described her mindless, thoughtless pattern of getting in the car and driving to fast-food restaurants and convenience stores for ice cream, cookies, and cakes. This was a pattern she had followed for many years—bingeing on large quantities of food for hours. The night of the overdose, Julie had simply had enough, and felt hopeless that she would ever be able to stop.

"I can't go on like this. I'm tired of fighting the cravings," were her first words to me.

I was astounded that she had become so helpless in her struggle with food cravings and binge eating that she would rather die. In that moment, I understood in a deeper way the magnitude of the problem of disordered appetite and how urgent it is that we find answers. Over the years, our understanding of food addiction has become grounded in neuroscience, and binge eating disorder has finally been established as a diagnosis requiring medical and psychological treatment.

In prehistoric times, animals developed complicated, redundant, and well-preserved mechanisms to store fat and protect themselves from starvation; mechanisms some have described as "Survival of the Fattest." Consuming sufficient food for energy metabolism is essential for the survival of all species in the animal kingdom. Mammalian brains have evolved several interrelated neural and biochemical systems that drive feeding behaviors. These strong evolutionary forces still propel our biological drives, despite the fact that modern environments bear little to no resemblance to those in which our ancient ancestors first evolved. In the modern world, the most potent driver of feeding behavior is its rewarding nature. Most of us are storing away fat for a famine that is not an imminent threat and will likely never come.

Not all of us, however, are driven by food cravings we cannot control. I hope you can appreciate how genetic variability leaves some individuals vulnerable to having their bodies' reward systems hijacked. Particular foods you eat, in combination with stress and an erratic pattern of restrictive eating and bingeing, send some of you on a one-way ride on the roller coaster, where you are buffeted wildly and no longer the driver of your own eating behaviors. As I learned so dramatically from Julie, stopping the cravings that fuel the roller coaster is a matter of life or death.

My search for an answer to appetite control did not lead me to a simple one. But it did lead me to a simple goal. I have learned that treatment for disordered appetite should focus on optimizing brain health. This means providing the body and brain with the essential nutrients that are necessary to regulate mood, emotion, behavior, and appetite. This is your New Hope.

Although the goal is simple and the same for everyone, the answer is complicated because we are all unique; not only in the way we look and in our past experiences, but also in our metabolism and biochemistry. No two individuals have exactly the same thumbprint, not even identical twins. Rather than being random, these differences usually result from predictable variations in genetics and in the interaction between our genes and the environment. In fact, one third of genetic variations are associated with the body's ability to utilize and absorb nutrients. These variations mean that every individual has unique metabolic needs and that the metabolism of essential nutrients varies among individuals.

Atop biochemical individuality lies another factor in this equation: the way in which each of us experiences food differs and is also wholly subjective. Food is not just about calories and energy for survival. Food is about cultural history, about connections and relationships. Food is about memories and family. The experience of tasting food floods our brains with memories from long ago that create an emotional landscape that is vivid, immediate, and often independent of logical thinking.

Food is about pleasure and our deepest feelings.

So, with the almost infinite variations in our life experience and biochemical individuality, common sense dictates there would not be a simple answer to binge eating. But there absolutely are answers—strategies that can be tailored to each unique individual. These answers are grounded in the field of integrative medicine, a therapeutic approach to healing based on biochemical individuality and the understanding that body, mind, and spirit are all interconnected. Rather than simply attempting to eliminate the symptoms of a disorder, integrative medicine aims to restore balance in the body by adjusting the factors—both internal and external—that nurture or repair the whole being. Both traditional and complementary therapies can be incorporated into an integrative approach.

When an individual's neurochemistry is disordered because of stress, genetics, inflammation, or malnutrition, disordered appetite and binge eating disorder are often present. Solutions to binge eating therefore involve regulating biochemistry. The New Hope model will help you optimize your brain health. With the brain's reward system no longer out of kilter, a healthy appetite returns. Moreover, appetite control will free you to lead a lively, unique life with the psychological freedom to be you.

Research has shown that parts of the brain associated with memory and desire are stimulated when someone addicted to food sees an image of, for example, a cheeseburger. We now know that MRIs reveal actual changes in the brains of people who have escaped the stranglehold of addiction. Marc Galanter MD, Professor of Psychiatry at NYU, has shown that when people share their individual stories of overcoming cravings or addiction in a supportive setting, the resulting activation of the dopamine reward system can be observed in in MRI scans. We can actually see in a concrete way the effects of an intangible process - such as emotional support - upon the physical structures of the brain.

The New Hope model represents real hope for overcoming binge eating and food addiction. I have seen thousands of patients break free of food cravings. More research into binge eating disorder and food addiction will offer new insights over time, but right now the New Hope model will empower you to change your relationship with food.

I wrote this book to offer a science-based approach to overcoming food cravings, food addiction, and chronic disordered eating patterns. The success achieved by patients who have followed this integrative model means that you, too, can move past the days and years that you have felt controlled by an appetite gone wild.

I am confident that the New Hope model will lead you to the most important hope of all: that you will be able to step off the roller coaster of disordered eating and reclaim your life.

Summary

In a modern world where food is entwined with nearly everything we do, the appetite that once served as a mechanism for survival can quickly become problematic. An appetite gone awry permeates all areas of one's life, from social interactions, mood, and emotional connections to the physical health of the immune, cardiovascular, and digestive systems. Food addiction and binge eating disorder are serious medical diagnoses that evolve when appetite spins out of control. Binge eating disorder is complex, pervasive, and impossible to resolve with logic or willpower alone. An effective treatment plan incorporates advanced medical and psychological approaches that are specifically tailored to one's unique biochemistry and experiences.

The New Hope model described in this book combines the best in traditional and complementary approaches for recovery from appetite disturbances, food addiction, and chronic binge eating. At the center of the New Hope model are targeted therapies that restore nutrient balance to heal the body and mind. When equipped with the necessary building blocks, the body is able to recover the innate biochemical stability that guides appropriate eating, making a healthy relationship with food possible. The New Hope model provides the tools you need to step off the roller coaster of disordered eating and take back control over your life.

Key Points

- Food addiction and binge eating disorder are serious neurological diagnoses that require a combination of medical and psychological treatment.
- In the modern world, the widespread availability of food and related media displays make navigating nutritional choices more difficult than ever.
- Food is not only consumed for survival; it is part of traditions, memories, pleasure, and our most intimate feelings.
- Smelling, tasting, seeing, or even just thinking about food can stimulate primal hunger cues that signal for us to eat more for "survival," even when it is not biologically necessary.
- An overwhelmed, malfunctioning appetite is at the base of food addiction and binge eating disorder.
- The successful treatment plan for disordered eating takes into account *all* of the factors that affect appetite, including biological, psychological, social, and cultural influences.
- Targeting the brain and nervous system with specific nutritional therapies can help restore appropriate appetite signals and stabilize the behaviors and emotions surrounding food.
- The New Hope model is an integrative approach to resolving food addiction and chronic binge eating that combines the best traditional and complementary therapies currently available.

- By focusing on the whole being, the New Hope model will empower you to step off the roller coaster of disordered eating and take back your life.

ABOUT THE AUTHORS

James M. Greenblatt, MD

A pioneer in the field of integrative medicine, James M. Greenblatt, MD, has treated patients with attention, mood, and eating disorders since 1988. After receiving his medical degree and fulfilling his psychiatry residency at George Washington University, Dr. Greenblatt completed a fellowship in child and adolescent psychiatry at Johns Hopkins Medical School. Dr. Greenblatt currently serves as the Chief Medical Officer at Walden Behavioral Care in Waltham, MA and serves as an Assistant Clinical Professor of Psychiatry at Tufts University School of Medicine and the Dartmouth College Geisel School of Medicine.

An acknowledged integrative medicine expert, educator, and author, Dr. Greenblatt has lectured internationally on the scientific evidence for nutritional interventions in psychiatry and mental illness. Through three decades of practice and research he has been a leading contributor to the revolution of patients and families seeking individualized care, and offers evidence-based approaches toward nuanced, integrative recovery.

In April of 2017 Dr. Greenblatt was inducted into the Orthomolecular Medicine Hall of Fame by the International Society of Orthomolecular Medicine, which has honored significant contributors to medical science who operate from the perspective of biochemical individuality and nutrition-based therapies since 2004. Dr. Greenblatt shares this distinction with recognized founders of the field of integrative medicine, including Abraham Hoffer, Linus Pauling, and Roger Williams.

Dr. Greenblatt's book series, *Psychiatry Redefined*, draws on his many years of experience as a practicing clinician and his expertise in the application of integrative medicine for psychiatry. His knowledge as to the myriad biologic and environmental factors that influence the development and manifestation of mental illness, as well as the way in which such factors interact to shape therapeutic trajectories, has made him a highly sought-after speaker who has lectured extensively at scientific conferences around the world. He currently offers online courses for professionals as well as specialized fellowship programs in functional medicine approaches to integrative psychiatry.

Information about the *Psychiatry Redefined* book series, *Psychiatry Redefined* educational opportunities, and upcoming events involving Dr. Greenblatt can be found at: www.jamesgreenblattmd.com.

Virginia Ross-Taylor, PhD

Virginia Ross Taylor is a freelance writer specializing in behavioral health and medicine. A native of Pittsburgh, she has an undergraduate degree from Duke and a PhD from Emory University. She now lives with her family outside Boston. She can be reached at virginiarosstaylor@verizon.net.

REFERENCES

Integrative Medicine for Binge Eating
References by Chapter

Introduction
Hallowell EM. *CrazyBusy: Overstretched, Overbooked and About to Snap! Strategies for Handling Your Fast-Paced Life.* New York, NY: Ballantine; 2007.

Higgins I. An open apology to all of my weight loss clients. *Huffington Post.* http://www.huffingtonpost.com/iris-higgins/an-open-apology-to-all-of_b_3762714.html. Published August 16 2013.

PART I: THE ROLLER COASTER RIDE OF BINGE EATING AND FOOD ADDICTION

Chapter 1 | The New Hope: Restoring Control

Avena N, Rada P, Koebel B. (2008). Evidence of sugar addiction: Behavioral and neurochemical effects of intermittent, excessive sugar intake. *Neurosci Biobehavi Rev.* 2008;32(1):20-39.

Colantuoni C, Schwenker J, McCarthy J et al. (2001). Excessive sugar intake alters binding to dopamine and mu-opioid receptors in the brain. *NeuroReport.* 2001;12(16):3549-3552.

Dagher A. The neurobiology of appetite: hunger as addiction. *Int J Obes (Lond).* 2009;*33*(Suppl 2): S30-33.

Gearhardt AN, Yokum S, Orr PT, Stice E, Corbin WR, Brownell KD. Neural correlates of food addiction. *Arch Gen Psychiatry.* 2011;68(8):808-816.

Holden JE, Jeong Y, Forrest JM. The endogenous opioid system and clinical pain management. *AACN Clin Issues.* 2005;16(3):291-301.

Ifland JR, Preuss, HG, Marcus MT et al. Refined food addiction: A classic substance use disorder. *Med Hypotheses.* 2009;72(5):518-526.

Rogers PJ, Smit HJ. (2000). Food craving and food "addiction": a critical review of the evidence from a biopsychosocial perspective. *Pharmacol Biochem Behav.* 2000;66(1):3-14.

Stice E, Yokum S, Blum K, Bohon C. Weight gain is associated with reduced striatal response to palatable food. *J Neurosci.* 2010;30(39):13105-13109.

Tellez LA, Medina S, Han W et al. A gut lipid messenger links excess dietary fat to dopamine deficiency. *Science.* 2013;341(6147):800-802.

Chapter 2 | Addicted to Food: My Dopamine Made Me Do It

Brzezinski M, Smith D. *Obsessed: America's Food Addiction and My Own.* New York, NY: Weinstein Books; 2013.

Cheren M, Foushi M, Gudmundsdotte, EH et al. Physical Craving and Food Addiction. *Sarasota, FL: The Food Addiction Institute; 2009.*

Davis C. A narrative review of binge eating and addictive behaviors: shared associations with seasonality and personality factors. *Front Psychiatry. 2013;4*: 183.

Gearhardt AN, Corbin WR, Brownell KD. Preliminary validation of the Yale Food Addiction Scale. *Appetite.* 2009;52(2):430-436.

Gearhardt AN, Grilo CM, DiLeone RJ, Brownell KD, Potenza MN. Can food be addictive? Public health and policy implications. *Addiction.* 2011;106(7):1208-1212.

Hyman SE. The neurobiology of addiction: Implications for voluntary control of behavior. *Am J Bioeth.* 2007;7(1):8-11.

Johnson PM, Kenny PJ. Dopamine D2 receptors in addiction-like reward dysfunction and compulsive eating in obese rats. *Nat Neurosci.* 2010;13(5):635-641.

Meule A. How prevalent is "food addiction"? *Front Psychiatry.* 2011;2: 61.

Moreno C, Tandon R. Should overeating and obesity be classified as an addictive disorder in DSM-5? *Curr Pharm Des.* 2011;17(12):1128-1131.

Parylak SL, Koob GF, Zorrilla EP. The dark side of food addiction. *Physiol Behav.* 2011;104(1):149-156.

Peeke P. *The hunger fix: The three-stage detox and recovery plan for overeating and food addiction.* New York, NY: Rodale Press; 2012.

Volkow ND, Fowler JS, Wang GJ, Baler R, Telang F. Imaging dopamine's role in drug abuse and addiction. *Neuropharmacology.* 2009;56(Suppl 1):3-8.

Volkow ND, O'Brien CP. Issues for DSM-5: Should obesity be included as a brain disorder? *Am J Psychiatry.* 2007;164(5):708-710.

Wang GJ, Volkow ND, Logan J et al. Brain dopamine and obesity. *The Lancet.* 2001;357(9253):354-357.

Weiner S. The addiction of overeating: Self-help groups as treatment models. *J Clin Psychol.* 1998;54(2):163-167.

Chapter 3 | The Appetite Gone Wild: Many Forms of Disordered Eating

Altarejos JY, Goebel N, Conkright MD et al. The Creb1 coactivator Crtc1 is required for energy balance and fertility. *Nat Med.* 2008;14(10):1112-1117.

American Psychiatric Association. *Diagnostic and statistical manual of mental disorders* (5th ed.). Arlington, VA: American Psychiatric Publishing; 2013.

Batterham RL, Cowley MA, Small CJ et al. Gut hormone PYY(3-36) physiologically inhibits food intake. *Nature.* 2002;418(6898):650-654.

Beck B, Stricker-Krongrad A, Nicolas JP, Burlet C. Chronic and continuous intracerebroventricular infusion of neuropeptide Y in Long-Evans rats mimics the feeding behaviour of obese Zucker rats. *Int J Obes Relat Metab Disord.* 1992;16(4):295-302.

Boswell T, Dunn IC, Corr SA. Hypothalamic neuropeptide Y mRNA is increased after feed restriction in growing broilers. *Poult Sci.* 1999;78(8):1203-1207.

Dryden S, Pickavance L, Frankish HM, Williams G. Increased neuropeptide Y secretion in the hypothalamic paraventricular nucleus of obese (*fa/fa*) Zucker rats. *Brain Res.* 1995;690(2):185-188.

Kinzl JF, Traweger C, Trefalt E, Mangweth B, Biebl W. Binge eating disorder in females: A population-based investigation. *Int J Eat Disord.* 1999;25(3):287-292.

Kotwal R, Kaneria R, Guerdjikova A. Binge-eating disorder: where medications fit in the comprehensive treatment of eating disturbance, obesity and depression. *Curr Psychiatr. 2004; 3*:31-47.

Leidy HJ, Racki EM. The addition of a protein-rich breakfast and its effects on acute appetite control and food intake in 'breakfast-skipping' adolescents. *Int J Obes.* 2010;34(7):1125-1133.

McKibbin PE, Rogers P, Williams G. Increased neuropeptide Y concentrations in the lateral hypothalamic area of the rat after the onset of darkness: possible relevance to the circadian periodicity of feeding behavior. *Life Sci.* 1991;48(26):2527-2533.

Volkow ND, Wang GJ, Baler RD. Reward, dopamine and the control of food intake: Implications for obesity. *Trends Cogn Sci.* 2011;15(1):37-46.

Chapter 4 | You Are Extraordinary: The Genetics of Appetite and Weight Control

Bahadir A, Eroz R, Dikici S. Investigation of MTHFR C677T gene polymorphism, biochemical and clinical parameters in Turkish migraine patients: association with allodynia and fatigue. *Cell Mol Neurobiol.* 2013;33(8):1055-1063.

Gilbody S, Lewis S, Lightfoot T. Methylenetetrahydrofolate reductase (MTHFR) genetic polymorphisms and psychiatric disorders: a HuGE review. *Am J Epidemiol.* 2006;165(1):1-13.

Guénard F, Deshaies Y, Cianflone K, Kral JG, Marceau P, Vohl MC. Differential methylation in glucoregulatory genes of offspring born before vs. after maternal gastrointestinal bypass surgery. *Proc Natl Acad Sci U S A.* 2012;110(28):11439-11444.

Hilbert A, Dierk JM, Conradt M et al. Causal attributions of obese men and women in genetic testing: implications of genetic/biological attributions. *Psychol Health.* 2009;24(7):749-761.

Javaras KN, Laird NM, Reichborn-Kjennerud T, Bulik CM, Hudson JI. Familiality and heritability of binge eating disorder: results of a case-control family study and a twin study. *Int J Eat Disord.* 2008;41(2):174-179.

Keller KL, Pietrobelli A, Must S, Faith MS. Genetics of eating and its relation to obesity. *Curr Atheroscler Rep.* 2002;4(3):176-182.

Lilenfeld LR, Ringham R, Kalarchian MA, Marcus MD. A family history study of binge-eating disorder. *Compr Psychiatry.* 2008;49(3):247-254.

Lumey LH, Stein AD, Kahn HS et al. Cohort Profile: the Dutch Hunger Winter Families Study. *Int J Epidemiol.* 2007;36(6):1196-1204.

Munn-Chernoff MA, Duncan AE, Grant JD et al. A twin study of alcohol dependence, binge eating and compensatory behaviors. *J Stud Alcohol and Drugs.* 2013;74(5):664-673.

Reichborn-Kjennerud T, Bulik CM, Tambs K, Harris JR. Genetic and environmental influences on binge eating in the absence of compensatory behaviors: a population-based twin study. *Int J Eat Disord.* 2003;36(3):307-314.

Trace SE, Baker JH, Peñas-Lledó E, Bulik CM. The genetics of eating disorders. *Annu Rev Clin Psychol.* 2013;9: 589-620.

Waterland RA, Jirtle RL. Transposable elements: targets for early nutritional effects on epigenetic gene regulation. *Mol Cell Biol.* 2003;23(15):5293-5300.

Williams RJ. *You Are Extraordinary.* New York, NY: Pyramid Books; 1967.

Chapter 5 | Comprehensive Evaluations for Appetite Control

Altman SE, Shankman SA. What is the association between obsessive–compulsive disorder and eating disorders? *Clin Psychol Rev.* 2009;29(7):638–646.

Anderluh MB, Tchanturia K, Rabe-Hesketh S, Treasure J. Childhood obsessive-compulsive personality traits in adult women with eating disorders: defining a broader eating disorder phenotype. *Am J Psychiatry.* 2003;160(2):242-247.

Brewerton TD. Eating disorders, trauma and comorbidity: focus on PTSD. *Eat Disord.* 2007;15(4):285-304.

Bulik CM, Sullivan PF, Fear JL, Joyce PR. Eating disorders and antecedent anxiety disorders: A controlled study. *Acta Psychiatr Scand.* 1997;96(2):101-107.

Courtney EA, Gamboz J, Johnson JG. Problematic eating behaviors in adolescents with low self-esteem and elevated depressive symptoms. *Eat Behav.* 2008;9(4):408–414.

Davis C, Curtis C, Levitan RD, Kaplan AS, Kennedy JL. Evidence that 'food addiction' is a valid phenotype of obesity. *Appetite.* 2011;57(3):711-717.

Davis C, Levitan RD, Smith M, Tweed S, Curtis C. Associations among overeating, overweight and attention deficit/hyperactivity disorder: a structural equation modeling approach. *Eat Behav.* 2006;7(3):266-274.

Davis C, Patte K, Levitan RD et al. A psycho-genetic study of associations between the symptoms of binge eating disorder and those of attention deficit (hyperactivity) disorder. *J Psychiatr Res.* 2009;43(7):687-696.

Farber SK. The last word: the comorbidity of eating disorders and attention-deficit hyperactivity disorder. *Eat Disord.* 2010;18(1):81-89.

Godart NT, Flament MF, Lecrubier Y, Jeammet P. Anxiety disorders in anorexia nervosa and bulimia nervosa: co-morbidity and chronology of appearance. *European Psychiatry.* 2000;15(1):38-45.

Hartmann AS, Rief W, Hilbert A. Laboratory snack food intake, negative mood and impulsivity in youth with ADHD symptoms and episodes of loss of control eating. Where is the missing link? *Appetite.* 2012;58(2):672-678.

Pallister E, Waller G. Anxiety in the eating disorders: understanding the overlap. *Clin Psychol Rev.* 2008;28(3):366–386.

Paxton SJ, Diggens J. Avoidance coping, binge eating and depression: an examination of the escape theory of binge eating. *Int J Eat Disord.* 1996;22(1):83-87.

Peterson RE, Latendresse SJ, Bartholome LT, Warren CS, Raymond NC. Binge eating disorder mediates links between symptoms of depression, anxiety and caloric intake in overweight and obese women. *J Obes. 2012*; 2012:407103.

Speranza M, Corcos M, Godart N et al. Obsessive compulsive disorders in eating disorders. *Eat Behav.* 2001;2(3):193-207.

Spoor ST, Stice E, Bekker MH, Van Strien T, Croon MA, Van Heck GL. Relations between dietary restraint, depressive symptoms and binge eating: a longitudinal study. *Int J Eat Disord.* 2006;39(8):700–707.

Van Strien T, van der Zwaluw C, Engels RC. Emotional eating in adolescents: a gene (SLC6A4/5-HTT)-depressive feelings interaction analysis. *J Psychiatr Res.* 2010;44(15):1035-1042.

Chapter 6 | Food Addiction: The Science of Sugar

Aronson M, Budhos M. *Sugar Changed the World: A Story of Magic, Spice, Slavery, Freedom and Science.* New York: Clarion Books; 2010.

Avena NM, Bocarsly ME, Rada P, Kim A, Hoebel BG. After daily bingeing on a sucrose solution, food deprivation induces anxiety and accumbens dopamine/acetylcholine imbalance. *Physiol Behav.* 2008;94(3):309-315.

Avena NM, Rada P, Hoebel BG. Evidence for sugar addiction: Behavioral and neurochemical effects of intermittent, excessive sugar intake. *Neurosci Biobehav Rev.* 2008;32(1):20-39.

Avena NM, Rada P, Hoebel BG. Sugar and fat bingeing have notable differences in addictive-like behavior. *J Nutr.* 2009;139(3):623-628.

Blumenthal DM, Gold MS. Neurobiology of food addiction. *Curr Opin Clin Nutr Metab Care.* 2010;13(4):359-365.

Colantuoni C, Rada P, McCarthy J et al. Evidence that intermittent, excessive sugar intake causes endogenous opioid dependence. *Obes Res.* 2002;10(6):478-488.

Jee SH, Ohrr H, Sull JW, Yun JE, Ji M, Samet JM. Fasting serum glucose levels and cancer risk in Korean men and women. *JAMA*. 2005;293(2):194-202.

Johnson R. *The Sugar Fix*. New York: Simon & Schuster; 2009.

Liu Y, von Deneen KM, Kobeissy FH, Gold MS. Food addiction and obesity: evidence from bench to bedside. *J Psychoactive Drugs*. 2010;42(2):133-145.

Lustig RH, Schmidt LA, Brindis CD. Public health: The toxic truth about sugar. *Nature*. 2012;482(7383):27-29.

Taubes G. *Good Calories, Bad Calories*. New York: Random House; 2008.

Taubes G, Couzens CK. Sweet little lies: the 40-year campaign to cover up evidence that sugar kills. *Mother Jones*. https://www.motherjones.com/environment/2012/10/sugar-industry-lies-campaign/. Published November/December 2012.

Volkow ND, Wise RA. How can drug addiction help us understand obesity? *Nat Neurosci*. 2005;8(5):555-560.

Wang GJ, Volkow ND, Logan J et al. Brain dopamine and obesity. *The Lancet*. 2001;357(9253):354-357.

Chapter 7 | Food Addiction: The Chemistry of Dairy and Wheat

Baltaci AK, Gokbel H, Mogulkoc R, Okudan N, Ucok K, Halifeoglu I. The effects of exercise and zinc deficiency on some elements in rats. *Biol Trace Elem Res*. 2010;134(1):79-83.

Cade R, Privette M, Fregly M et al. Autism and schizophrenia: intestinal disorders. *Nutr Neurosci*. 2010;3(1):57-72.

Christie MJ. Cellular neuroadaptations to chronic opioids: tolerance, withdrawal and addiction. *Br J Pharmacol*. 2008;154(2):384-396.

Davis W. *Wheat Belly*. New York, NY: Rodale Books; 2011.

De Noni I, FitzGerald RJ, Korhonen HJT et al. Review of the potential health impact of β-casomorphins and related peptides. *European Food Safety Authority Scientific Report*. 2009; 231:1-107.

Dohan FC. More on celiac disease as a model for schizophrenia. *Biol Psychiatry*. 1983;18(5):561-4.

Froehlich, J. Opioid peptides. *Alcohol Health Res World.* 1997;21(2):132-136.

Gable RS. Toward a comparative overview of dependence potential and acute toxicity of psychoactive substances used nonmedically. *Am J Drug Alcohol Abuse.* 1993;19(3):263-281.

Gillberg C, Terenius L, Lönnerholm G. Endorphin activity in childhood psychosis: Spinal fluid levels in 24 cases. *Arch Gen Psychiatry.* 1985;42(8):780-783.

Hellzén M, Larsson JO, Reichelt KL, Rydelius PA. Urinary peptide levels in women with eating disorders. A pilot study. *Eating Weight Disord.* 2003;8(1):55-61.

Hole K, Lingjaerde O, Mørkrid L et al. Attention deficit disorders: a study of peptide-containing urinary complexes. *J Dev Behav Pediatr.* 1988;9(4):205-212.

Hole K, Bergslien H, Jørgensen HA, Berge OG, Reichelt KL, Trygstad OE. A peptide-containing fraction in the urine of schizophrenic patients which stimulates opiate receptors and inhibits dopamine uptake. *Neuroscience.* 1979;4(12):1883-1893.

Kamiński S, Cieslińska A, Kostyra E. Polymorphism of bovine beta-casein and its potential effect on human health. *J Appl Genet.* 2007;48(3):189–198.

Knivsberg AM. Urine patterns, peptide levels and IgA/IgG antibodies to food proteins in children with dyslexia. *Pediatr Rehabil.* 1997;1(1):25-33.

Levy SE, Souders MC, Ittenbach RF, Giarelli E, Mulberg AE, Pinto-Martin JA. Relationship of dietary intake to gastrointestinal symptoms in children with autistic spectrum disorders. *Biol Psychiatry.* 2007;61(4):492-497.

Lindström LH, Nyberg F, Terenius L et al. CSF and plasma beta-casomorphin-like opioid peptides in postpartum psychosis. *Am J Psychiatry.* 1984;141(9):1059-1066.

Pedersen OS, Liu Y, Reichelt KL. Serotonin uptake stimulating peptide found in plasma of normal individuals and in some autistic urines. *J Pept Res.* 1999;53(6):641-646.

Perlmutter D. *Grain Brain*. New York, NY: Little, Brown and Company; 2013.

Reichelt KL. Peptides as carriers of information in psychiatric diseases. *Nord Med.* 1980;95(11):283-6.

Reichelt KL, Knivsberg AM. Can the pathophysiology of autism be explained by the nature of the discovered urine peptides? *Nutr Neurosci.* 2003;6(1):19-28.

Reichelt KL, Knivsberg AM. The possibility and probability of gut-to-brain connection in autism. *Ann Clin Psychiatry.* 2009;21(4):205-211.

Reichelt KL, Stensrud M. Increase in urinary peptides prior to the diagnosis of schizophrenia. *Schizophr Res.* 1998;34(3):211-213.

Rossetti ZL, Melis F, Carboni S, Gessa GL. Dramatic depletion of mesolimbic extracellular dopamine after withdrawal from morphine, alcohol or cocaine: a common neurochemical substrate for drug dependence. *Ann NY Acad Sci.* 2006; 654:513–516.

Saelid G, Haug JO, Heiberg T, Reichelt KL. Peptide-containing fractions in depression. *Biol Psychiatry.* 1985;20(3):245-256.

Severance EG, Dupont D, Dickerson FB et al. Immune activation by casein dietary antigens in bipolar disorder. *Bipolar Disord.* 2010;12(8):834–842.

Sun Z, Cade R. A peptide found in schizophrenia and autism causes behavioral changes in rats. *Autism.* 1999;3(1):85-95.

PART II: PERSONALIZED NUTRITIONAL SUPPLEMENTS FOR BINGE EATING AND FOOD ADDICTION

Chapter 8 | Laboratory Evaluations for Individualized Nutritional Support

Almeida OP, McCaul K, Hankey GJ, Norman P, Jamrozik K, Flicker L. Homocysteine and depression in later life. *Arch Gen Psychiatry.* 2008;65(11):1286-1294.

Amr M, El-Mogy A, Shams T, Vieira K, Lakhan SE. Efficacy of vitamin C as an adjunct to fluoxetine therapy in pediatric major depressive disorder: a randomized, double-blind, placebo-controlled pilot study. *Nutr J.* 2013; 12:31.

Bland J. Systems biology, functional medicine and folates. *Altern Ther Health Med.* 2008;14(3):18-20.

Bottiglieri T. Folate, vitamin B12, and S-adenosylmethionine. *Psychiatr Clin North Am.* 2013;36(1):1-13.

Brown AS, Sourander A, Hinkka-Yli-Salomäki S, McKeague IW, Sundvall J, Surcel HM. Elevated maternal C-reaction protein and autism in a national birth cohort. *Mol Psychiatry.* 2014;19(2):259-264.

De Heredia FP, Cerezo D, Zamora S, Garaulet M. Effect of dehydroepiandrosterone on protein and fat digestibility, body protein and muscular composition in high-fat-diet-fed old rats. *Br J Nutr.* 2007;97(3):464-470.

Fiedorowicz JG, Haynes WG. Cholesterol, mood and vascular health: untangling the relationship: does low cholesterol predispose to depression and suicide, or vice versa? *Curr Psychiatr.* 2010;9(7):17-A.

Guerrera MP, Volpe SL, Mao JJ. Therapeutic uses of magnesium. *Am Fam Physician.* 2009;80(2):157-162.

Halford JC, Harrold JA. 5-HT(2C) receptor agonists and the control of appetite. *Handb Exp Pharmacol.* 2012; 209:349-356.

Littarru GP, Tiano L. Clinical aspects of coenzyme Q10: an update. *Curr Opin Clin Nutr Metab Care.* 2005;8(6):641-646.

Lord RS, Bralley JA, eds. *Laboratory evaluations for integrative and functional medicine.* Duluth, GA: Metametrix Institute; 2008.

Lukaczer, D, Schiltz B. Assessment and therapeutic strategy—a place to start. In: Jones DS, ed. *Textbook of functional medicine.* Gig Harbor, WA: Institute for Functional Medicine; 2005: pp. 706-708.

Maninger N, Wolkowitz OM, Reus VI, Epel ES, Mellon SH. Neurobiological and Neuropsychiatric Effects of Dehydroepiandrosterone (DHEA) and DHEA Sulfate (DHEAS). *Front Neuroendocrinol.* 2009;30(1):65-91.

Melanson KJ, Angelopoulos TJ, Nguyen V, Zukley L, Lowndes J, Rippe JM. High-fructose corn syrup, energy intake and appetite regulation. *Am J Clin Nutr.* 2008;88(6):1738S-1744S.

Mizuno K, Tanaka M, Nozaki S et al. Antifatigue effects of coenzyme Q10 during physical fatigue. *Nutrition.* 2008;24(4):293-299.

Patrick RP, Ames BN. Vitamin D hormone regulates serotonin synthesis. Part I: relevance for autism. *FASEB J.* 2014;28(6):2398-2413.

Raj YP. Treating thyroid disorders and depression: 3 case studies. *Curr Psychiatr.* 2013;12(1):17-21.

Romero-Corral A, Sierra-Johnson J, Lopez-Jimenez F et al. Relationships between leptin and C-reactive protein with cardiovascular disease in the adult general population. *Nat Clin Pract Cardiovasc Med.* 2008;5(7):418-425.

Rondanelli M, Klersy C, Iadarola P, Monteferrario F, Opizzi A. Satiety and amino-acid profile in overweight women after a new treatment using a natural plant extract sublingual spray formulation. *Int J Obes (Lond).* 2009;33(10):1174-1182.

Sahley BJ. *Weight Control and Amino Acids.* New York, NY: Pain & Stress Publications; 2010.

Swenne I, Rosling A, Tengblad S, Vessby B. Omega-3 polyunsaturated essential fatty acids are associated with depression in adolescents with eating disorders and weight loss. *Acta Paediatr.* 2011;100(12):1610-1615.

Vahdat Shariatpanaahi M, Vahdat Shariatpanaahi Z, Moshtaaghi M, Shahbaazi SH, Abadi A. The relationship between depression and serum ferritin level. *Eur J Clin Nutr.* 2007;61(4):532-535.

Xu Y, Nedungadi TP, Zhu L et al. Distinct hypothalamic neurons mediate estrogenic effects on energy homeostasis and reproduction. *Cell Metab.* 2011;14(4):453-465.

Chapter 9 | Controlling Appetite with Amino Acid Supplements

Ballinger AB, Clark ML. L-phenylalanine releases cholecystokinin (CCK) in association with reduced food intake in humans:

evidence for a physiological role of CCK in control of eating. *Metabolism.* 1994;43(6):735-738.

Baranowski B, Wolinsla-Witort E, Wasilewska-Dziubinska E, Roguski K, Martynska L, Chmielowska M. (2003). The role of neuropeptides in the disturbed control of appetite and hormone secretion on eating disorders. *Neuro Endocrinol Lett.* 2003;24(6):431-434.

Birdsall TC. 5-Hydroxytryptophan: a clinically-effective serotonin precursor. *Altern Med Rev.* 1998;3(4):271-280.

Cangiano C, Ceci F, Cairella M et al. The effects of 5-hydroxytryptophan on eating behavior and adherence to dietary prescriptions in obese adult subjects. *Adv Exp Med Biol.* 1991; 294:591-593.

Cangiano C, Ceci F, Cascino A et al. Eating behavior and adherence to dietary prescriptions in obese adult subjects treated with 5-hydroxytryptophan. *Am J Clin Nutr.* 1992;56(5):863-867.

Ceci F, Cangiano C, Cariella M et al. The effects of oral 5-hydroxytryptophan administration on feeding behavior in obese adult female subjects. *J Neural Transm.* 1989;76(2):109-117.

Crayhon R. *The Carnitine Miracle.* Lanham, MD: Ronan & Littefield; 1998.

Cynober L. Ornitine alpha-ketoglutarate as a potent precursor of arginine and nitric oxide: a new job for an old friend. *J Nutr.* 2004;134(10 Suppl):2858S-2862S.

Dhillo WS. Appetite regulation: an overview. *Thyroid.* 2007;17(5):433-445.

Erdmann R. *The Amino Revolution.* New York: Simon & Schuster; 1987.

Fernstrom JD. Dietary effects on brain serotonin synthesis: relationship to appetite regulation. *Am J Clin Nutr.* 1985;42(5 Suppl):1072-1082.

Furuse M, Choi YH, Yang SI, Kita K, Okumura J. Enhanced release of cholecystokinin in chickens fed diets high in phenylalanine or tyrosine. *Comp Biochem Physiol.* 1992;99(3):449-451.

Goldbloom DS, Garfinkel PE, Katz R, Brown GM. The hormonal response to intravenous 5-hydroxytryptophan in bulimia nervosa. *J Psychosom Res.* 1996;40(3):289-297.

Goldstone, T. Hormone ghrelin raises desire for high-calorie foods. Talk presented at: The Endocrine Society's 92nd Annual Meeting and Expo; June 19-22, 2010; San Diego, CA.

Hao S, Avraham Y, Bonne O, Berry EM. Separation-induced body weight loss, impairment in alteration behavior: effects of tyrosine. *Pharmacol Biochem Behav.* 2001;68(2):273-281.

Jimerson DC, Wolfe BE. Neuropeptides in eating disorders. *CNS Spectr.* 2004;9(7):516-522.

Jobgen W, Meininger CJ, Jobgen SC et al. Dietary L-arginine supplementation reduces white fat gain and enhances skeletal muscle-bound fat masses in diet-induced obese rats. *J Nutr.* 2009;139(2):230-237.

Pagoto SL, Spring B, McChargue D et al. Acute tryptophan depletion and sweet food consumption by overweight adults. *Eat Behav.* 2009;10(1):36-41.

Pohle-Krausa RJ, Navia JL, Madore EY, Nyrop JE, Pelkman CL. Effects of L-phenylalanine on energy intake on overweight and obese women's interaction with dietary restraint status. *Appetite.* 2008;51(1):111-119.

Rondanelli M, Klersy C, Iadarola P, Monteferrario F, Opizzi A. Satiety and amino-acid profile in overweight women after a new treatment using a natural plant extract sublingual spray formulation. *Int J Obes (Lond).* 2009;33(10):1174-1182.

Sugino T, Shirai T, Kajimoto Y, Kajimoto O. L-ornithine supplementation attenuates physical fatigue in healthy volunteers by modulating lipid and amino acid metabolism. *Nutr Res.* 2008;28(11):738-743.

Welzin TE, Fernstrom MH, Kaye WH. Serotonin and bulimia. *Nutr Rev.* 1994;52(12):399-408.

Wurtman RJ, Wurtman JJ, Regan MM, McDermott JM, Tsay RH, Beau JJ. Effects of normal meals rich in carbohydrates or proteins on plasma tryptophan and tyrosine rates. *Am J Clin Nutr.* 2003;77(1):128-132.

Yoshiji H, Noguchi R, Kitade M et al. Branched-chain amino acids suppress insulin-resistance-based hepatocarcinogenesis in obese diabetic rats. *J Gastroenterol.* 2009;44(5):483-491.

Zemel MB, Bruckbauer A. Effects of a leucine and pyridoxine-containing nutraceutical on body weight and composition in obese subjects. *Diabetes Metab Syndr Obes.* 2013; 6:309-315.

Chapter 10 | Controlling Appetite with Vitamin and Mineral Supplements

Abou-Saleh MT, Coppen A. Serum and red blood cell folate in depression. *Acta Psychiatr Scand.* 1989;80(1):78-82.

Barragan-Rodriguez L, Rodriguez-Moran M, Guerreo-Romero F. Efficacy and safety of oral magnesium supplementation in the treatment of depression in the elderly with type 2 diabetes: a randomized, equivalent trial. *Magnesium Res.* 2008;21(4):218-223.

Benjamin J, Levine J, Fux M, Aviv A, Levy D, Belmaker RH. Double-blind, placebo-controlled, crossover trial of inositol treatment for panic disorder. *Am J Psychiatry.* 1995;152(7):1084-1086.

Beydoun MA, Fanelli Kuczmarski MT, Beydoun HA et al. The sex-specific role of plasma folate in mediating the association of dietary quality with depressive symptoms. *J Nutr.* 2010;140(2):338-347.

Ciacci C, Peluso G, Iannoni E et al. L-carnitine in the treatment of fatigue in adult celiac disease patients: a pilot study. *Dig Liver Dis.* 2007;39(10):922-928.

Colodny L, Hoffman RL. Inositol—Clinical applications for exogenous use. *Altern Med Rev.* 1998;3(6):432-447.

Coppen A. Bailey J. Enhancement of the antidepressant action of fluoxetine by folic acid: a randomized, placebo-controlled trial. *J Affect Disord.* 2000;60(2):121-130.

Cruciani RA, Dvorkin E, Homel P et al. Safety, tolerability and symptom outcomes associated with L-carnitine supplementation in patients with cancer, fatigue and carnitine deficiency: a phase I/II study. *J Pain Symptom Manage.* 2006;32(6):551-559.

Davidson JR, Abraham K, Connor KM, McLeod MN. Effectiveness of chromium in atypical depression: a placebo-controlled trial. *Biol Psychiatry.* 2003;53(3):261-264.

Docherty JP, Sack DA, Roffman M, Finch M, Komorowski JR. A double-blind, placebo-controlled, exploratory trial of chromium picolinate in atypical depression: effect on carbohydrate craving. *J Psychiatr Pract.* 2005;11(5):302-314.

Eby GA, Eby KL. Rapid recovery from major depression using magnesium treatment. *Med Hypotheses*. 2006;67(2):362-370.

Fava M, Mischoulon D. Folate in depression: Efficacy, safety differences in formulations and clinical issues. *J Clin Psychiatry*. 2009;70(Suppl 5):12-17.

Fava M, Borus JS, Alpert JE, Nierenberg AA, Rosenbaum JF, Bottiglieri T. Folate, vitamin B12 and homocysteine in major depressive disorder. *Am J Psychiatry*. 1997;154(3):426-428.

Ford ES, Mokdad AH. Dietary magnesium intake in a national sample of U.S. adults. *J Nutr*. 2003;133(9):2879-2882.

Fux M, Benjamin J, Belmaker RH. Inositol versus placebo augmentation of serotonin reuptake inhibitors in the treatment of obsessive-compulsive disorder: a double-blind cross-over study. *Int J Neuropsychopharmacol*. 1999;2(3):193-195.

Hansen CR Jr., Malecha M, Mackenzie TB, Kroll J. Copper and zinc deficiencies in association with depression and neurological findings. *Biol Psychiatry*. 1983;18(3):395-401.

Hintikka J, Tolmunen T, Tanskanen A, Viinamäki H. High vitamin B12 level and good treatment outcome may be associated in major depressive disorder. *BMC Psychiatry*. 2003; 3:17.

Jacka FN, Overland S, Stewart R, Tell GS, Bjelland I, Mykletun A. Association between magnesium intake and depression and anxiety in community-dwelling adults: the Hordaland health study. *Aust N Z J Psychiatry*. 2009;43(1):45-52.

Kishi T, Watanabe T, Folkers K. Bioenergetics in clinical medicine XV. Inhibition of coenzyme Q10-enzymes by clinically used adrenergic blockers of beta-receptors. *Res Commun Mol Pathol Pharmacol*. 1977;17(1):157-164.

Levenson CW. Zinc: the new antidepressant? *Nutr Rev*. 2006;64(1):39-42.

Maes M, D'Haese PC, Scharpé S, D'Hondt P, Cosyns P, De Broe ME. Hypozincemia in depression. *J Affect Disord*. 1994;31(2):135-140.

Maes M, Vandoolaeghe E, Neels, H et al. Lower serum zinc in major depression is a sensitive marker of treatment resistance of the immune/inflammatory response in that illness. *Biol Psychiatry*. 1997;42(5):349-358.

Malaguarnera M, Cammalleri L, Gargante MP, Vacante M, Colonna V, Motta M. L-carnitine treatment reduces severity of physical and mental fatigue and increases cognitive functions in centenarians: a randomized and controlled clinical trial. *Am J Clin Nutr*. 2007;86(6):1738-1744.

Mamalakis G, Tornaritis M, Kafatos A. Depression and adipose essential polyunsaturated fatty acids. *Prostaglandins Leukot Essent Fatty Acids*. 2002;67(5):311-318.

McLeod MN, Golden RN. Chromium treatment of depression. *Int J Neuropsychopharmacol*. 2000;3(4):311-314.

McLoughlin IJ, Hodge JS. Zinc in depressive disorder. *Acta Psychiatr Scand*. 1990;82(6):451-453.

Milaneschi Y, Shardell M, Corsi AM et al. Serum 25-hydroxyvitamin D and depressive symptoms in older women and men. *J Clin Endocrinol Metab*. 2010;95(7):3225-3233.

Mizuno K, Tanaka M, Nozaki S et al. Antifatigue effects of coenzyme Q10 during physical fatigue. *Nutrition*. 2004;24(4):293-299.

Morris MC, Evans DA, Bienias JL et al. Dietary folate and vitamin B12 intake and cognitive decline among community-dwelling older persons. *Arch Neurol*. 2005;62(4):641-645.

Morris MS, Jacques PF, Rosenberg IH, Selhub J. Folate and vitamin B-12 status in relation to anemia, macrocytosis and cognitive impairment in older Americans in the age of folic acid fortification. *Am J Clin Nutr*. 2007;85(1):193-200.

Narang RL, Gupta KR, Narang AP, Singh R. Levels of copper and zinc in depression. *Indian J Physiol Pharmacol*. 1991;35(4):272-274.

Nowak G, Siwek M, Dudek D, Zieba A, Pilc A. Effect of zinc supplementation on antidepressant therapy in unipolar depression: a preliminary placebo-controlled trial. *Pol J Pharmacol*. 2003;55(6):1143-1147.

Nowak G, Szewczyk B, Pilc A. Zinc and depression. An update. *Pharmacol Rep*. 2005;57(6):713-718.

Otto SJ, de Groot RH, Hornstra G. Increased risk of postpartum depressive symptoms is associated with slower normalization after pregnancy of the functional docosahexaenoic acid status. *Prostaglandins Leukot Essent Fatty Acids*. 2003;69(4):237-243.

Palatnik A, Frolov K, Fux M, Benjamin J. Double-blind, controlled, crossover trial of inositol versus fluvoxamine for the treatment of panic disorder. *J Clin Psychopharmacol*. 2001;21(3):335-339.

Papakostas GI, Petersen T, Mischoulon D et al. Serum folate, vitamin B12 and homocysteine in major depressive disorder, Part 2: predictors of relapse during the continuation phase of pharmacotherapy. *J Clin Psychiatry*. 2004;65(8):1096-1098.

Plioplys AV, Plioplys S. Amantadine and L-carnitine treatment of chronic fatigue syndrome. *Neuropsychobiology*. 1997;35(1):16-23.

Preuss G, Anderson RA. Chromium update: examining recent literature 1997-1998. *Curr Opin Clin Nutr Metab Care*. 1998;1(6):509-512.

Russ CS, Chrisley BM, Hendricks TA. Vitamin B6 status of depressed and obsessive-compulsive patients. *Nutr Rep Int*. 1983;27(4):867-873.

Sawada T, Yokoi K. Effect of zinc supplementation on mood states in young women: a pilot study. *Eur J Clin Nutr*. 2010;64(3):331-333.

Siwek M, Dudek D, Paul IA et al. Zinc supplementation augments efficacy of imipramine in treatment resistant patients: a double-blind, placebo-controlled study. *J Affect Disord*. 2009;118(1-3):187-195.

Stewart JW, Harrison W, Quitkin F, Baker H. Low B6 levels in depressed outpatients. *Biol Psychiatry*. 1984;19(4):613-616.

Sublette ME, Hibbeln JR, Galfalvy H, Oquendo MA, Mann JJ. Omega-3 polyunsaturated essential fatty acid status as a predictor of future suicide risk. *Am J Psychiatry*. 2006;163(6):1100-1102.

Szewczyk B, Poleszak E, Sowa-Kućma M et al. Antidepressant activity of zinc and magnesium in view of the current hypotheses of antidepressant action. *Pharmacol Rep*. 2008;60(5):588-599.

Tassabehji NM, Corniola RS, Alshingiti A, Levenson CW. Zinc deficiency induces depression-like symptoms in adult rats. *Physiol Behav*. 2008;95(3):365-369.

Tiemeier H, van Tuijl HR, Hofman A, Meijer J, Kiliaan AJ, Breteler MM. Vitamin B12, folate and homocysteine in depression: the Rotterdam Study. *Am J Psychiatry*. 2002;159(12):2099-2101.

Wójcik J, Dudek D, Schlegel-Zawadzka M et al. Antepartum/postpartum depressive symptoms and serum zinc and magnesium levels. *Pharmacol Rep*. 2006;58(4):571-576.

PART III: MEDICATIONS FOR BINGE EATING AND FOOD ADDICTION

Chapter 11 | Controlling Appetite with Medications

Arbaizar B, Gómez-Acebo I, Llorca J. Efficacy of topiramate in bulimia nervosa and binge-eating disorder: a systematic review. *Gen Hosp Psychiatry*. 2008;30(5):471-475.

Cassels C. Nasal spray shows promise for binge eating disorder. *Medscape.com*. https://www.medscape.com/viewarticle/805004. Published May 30 2013.

Claudino AM, de Oliveira IR, Appolinario JC et al. Double-blind, randomized, placebo-controlled trial of topiramate plus cognitive-behavior therapy in binge-eating disorder. *J Clin Psychiatry*. 2007;68(9):1324-1332.

Fleming JW, McClendon KS, Riche DM. New obesity agents: lorcaserin and phentermine/topiramate. *Ann Pharmacother*. 2013;47(7-8):1007-1016.

Gadde KM, Allison DB, Ryan DH et al. Effects of low-dose, controlled-release phentermine plus topiramate combination on weight and associated comorbidities in overweight and obese adults (CONQUER): a randomized, placebo-controlled, phase 3 trial. *The Lancet*. 2011;377(9774):1341-1352.

Gadde KM, Yonish GM, Foust MS, Wagner HR. Combination therapy of zonisamide and bupropion for weight reduction in obese women: a randomized, open-label study. *J Clin Psychiatry*. 2007;68(8):1226-1229.

Hansen K. *Brain Over Binge: Why I Was Bulimic, Why Conventional Therapy Didn't Work and How I Recovered for Good.* Phoenix, AZ: Camellia Publishing; 2011.

Hudson JI, McElroy SL, Raymond NC et al. Fluvoxamine in the treatment of binge-eating disorder: A multicenter, placebo-controlled, double-blind trial. *Am J Psychiatry.* 1998;155(12):1756-1762.

Husted DS, Shapira NA. Binge-eating disorder and new pharmacologic treatments. *Prim Psychiatry.* 2005;12(4):46-51.

Jonas JM, Gold MS. The use of opiate antagonists in treating bulimia: a study of low-dose versus high-dose naltrexone. *Psychiatry Res.* 1987;24(2):195-199.

Landabaso MA, Iraurgi I, Jimenez-Lerma JM et al. A randomized trial of adding fluoxetine to a naltrexone treatment programme for heroin addicts. *Addiction.* 1998;93(5):739-744.

Leaf C. Do clinical trials work? *The New York Times.* https://www.nytimes.com/2013/07/14/opinion/sunday/do-clinical-trials-work.html. Published July 13 2013.

Maremmani I, Marini G, Castrogiovanni P, Deltito J. The effectiveness of the combination fluoxetine-naltrexone in bulimia nervosa. *Eur Psychiatry.* 1996;11(6):322-324.

McElroy SL, Arnold LM, Shapira NA et al. Topiramate in the treatment of binge eating disorder associated with obesity: a randomized, placebo-controlled trial. *Am J Psychiatry.* 2003;160(2):255-261.

McElroy SL, Guerdjikova AI, Mori N, O'Melia AM. Pharmacological management of binge eating disorder: current and emerging treatment options. *Ther Clin Risk Manag.* 2012; 8:219-241.

McElroy SL, Guerdjikova AI, Martens B, Keck PE Jr., Pope HG, Hudson JI. Role of antiepileptic drugs in the management of eating disorders. *CNS Drugs.* 2009;23(2):139-56.

McElroy SL, Hudson JI, Capece JA et al. Topiramate in the treatment of binge eating disorder associated with obesity: a randomized, placebo-controlled trial. *Biol Psychiatry.* 2007;61(9):1039-1048.

McElroy SL, Hudson JI, Gasior M et al. Time course of the effects of lisdexamfetamine dimesylate in two phase 3, randomized, double-blind, placebo-controlled trials in adults with binge-eating disorder. *Int J Eat Disord.* 2017;50(8):884-892.

Milano W, Petrella C, Sabatino C, Capasso A. Treatment of bulimia nervosa with sertraline: a randomized controlled trial. *Adv Ther.* 2004;21(4):232-237.

Neumeister A, Winkler A, Wöber-Bingöl C. Addition of naltrexone to fluoxetine in the treatment of binge eating disorder. *Am J Psychiatry.* 1999;156(5):797.

Opioid antagonist naloxone nasal spray treatment for patients with binge eating disorder (BED): a randomized, controlled trial. Paper presented at the 166th annual meeting of the American Psychiatric Association; San Francisco, CA. May 2013.

Rueda-Clausen CF, Padwal RS, Sharma AM. New pharmacological approaches for obesity management. *Nat Rev Endocrinol.* 2013;9(8):467-478.

Shapira NA, Goldsmith TD, McElroy SL. Treatment of binge-eating disorder with topiramate: a clinical case series. *J Clin Psychiatry.* 2000;61(5):368-372.

Shapiro JR, Berkman ND, Brownley KA, Sedway JA, Lohr KN, Bulik CM. Bulimia nervosa treatment: a systematic review of randomized controlled trials. *Int J Eat Disord.* 2007;40(4):321-336.

Sinclair JD. Evidence about the use of naltrexone and different ways of using it in the treatment of alcoholism. *Alcohol Alcohol.* 2001;36(1):2-10.

Vyvanse approved for binge-eating disorder: how it works, benefits, & risks. *Mentalhealthdaily.com.* https://mentalhealthdaily.com/2015/02/06/vyvanse-approved-for-binge-eating-disorder-how-it-works-benefits-risks/. Published February 2015.

PART IV: LIFESTYLE CHANGES FOR BINGE EATING AND FOOD ADDICTION

Chapter 12 | What Not to Eat: High Fructose Corn Syrup & Artificial Sweeteners

Avena NM, Bocarsly ME, Rada P, Kim A, Hoebel BG. After daily bingeing on a sucrose solution, food deprivation induces anxiety and accumbens dopamine/acetylcholine imbalance. *Physiol Behav.* 2008;94(3):309-315.

Avena NM, Rada P, Hoebel BG. Evidence for sugar addiction: behavioral and neurochemical effects of intermittent, excessive sugar intake. *Neurosci Biobehav Rev.* 2008;32(1):20-39.

Basciano H, Federico L, Adeli K. Fructose, insulin resistance and metabolic dyslipidemia. *Nutr Metab (Lond).* 2005;2(1):5.

Bray GA. Fructose: Should we worry? *Int J Obes (Lond).* 2008;32(Suppl 7): S127-S131.

Brow, CM, Dulloo AG, Montani JP. Sugary drinks in the pathogenesis of obesity and cardiovascular diseases. *Int J Obes (Lond).* 2008;32(Suppl 6): S28-S34.

Centers for Disease Control and Prevention. Evaluation of consumer complaints related to aspartame use. *MMWR Morb Mortal Wkly Rep.* 1984;33(43):605-607.

Colantuoni C, Rada P, McCarthy J et al. Evidence that intermittent, excessive sugar intake causes endogenous opioid dependence. *Obes Res.* 2002;10(6):478-488.

Green E, Murphy C. Altered processing of sweet taste in the brain of diet soda drinkers. *Physiol Behav.* 2012;107(4):560-567.

Johnson PM, Kenny PJ. Dopamine D2 receptors in addiction-like reward dysfunction and compulsive eating in obese rats. *Nat Neurosci.* 2010;13(5):635-641.

Johnson R. *The Sugar Fix.* New York, NY: Simon & Schuster; 2008.

Lenoir M, Serre F, Cantin L, Ahmed SH. Intense sweetness surpasses cocaine reward. *PLoS ONE. 2007;2*(8): e698.

Lim JS, Mietus-Snyder M, Valente A, Schwartz JM, Lustig, RH. The role of fructose in the pathogenesis of NAFLD and the metabolic syndrome. *Nat Rev Gastroenterol Hepatol.* 2010;7(5):251-264.

Mattes RD, Popkin BM. Nonnutritive sweetener consumption in humans: effects on appetite and food intake and their putative mechanisms. *Am J Clin Nutr.* 2009;89(1):1-14.

Mayo Clinic Staff. Artificial sweeteners and other sugar substitutes. *Mayoclinic.com.* Retrieved from http://www.mayoclinic.com/health/artificial-sweeteners/MY00073. Published September 25 2018.

Morris NP. Hooked on diet soda: an addict tries to cut back because of its health hazards. *Bostonglobe.com.* https://www.bostonglobe.com/opinion/2013/08/10/america-diet-soda-addiction-health-hazard-can/v5TscM41c9NvboXtkhdCnI/story.html. Published August 11 2013.

Shapiro A, Mu W, Roncal C, Cheng KY, Johnson RJ, Scarpace PJ. Fructose-induced leptin resistance exacerbates weight gain in response to subsequent high-fat feeding. *Am J Physiol.* 2008;295(5): R1370-R1375.

Volkow ND, Wise RA. How can drug addiction help us understand obesity? *Nat Neurosci.* 2005;8(5):555-560.

Chapter 13 | What Not to Eat: Monosodium Glutamate

Andreazzi AE, Grassiolli S, Marangon PB et al. Impaired symphoadrenal axis function contributes to enhanced insulin secretion in prediabetic obese rats. *Exp Diabetes Res.* 2011; 2011:947917.

Beauchamp GK. Sensory and receptor responses to umami: an overview of pioneering work. *Am J Clin Nutr.* 2009;90(3):723S-727S.

Bellisle F. Experimental studies of food choices and palatability responses in European subjects exposed to the umami taste. *Asia Pac J Clin Nutr.* 2008;17(Suppl 1):376-379.

Blaylock RL. *Excitotoxins: The taste that kills.* Santa Barbara, CA: Health Press; 1997.

Castrogiovanni D, Gaillard RC, Giovambattista A, Spinedi E. Neuroendocrine, metabolic and immune functions during the acute phase response of inflammatory stress in monosodium l-glutamate-damaged, hyperadipose male rat. *Neuroendocrinology.* 2008;88(3):227-234.

Chevassus H, Renard E, Bertrand G et al. Effects of oral monosodium (L)-glutamate on insulin secretion and glucose tolerance in healthy volunteers. *Br J Clin Pharmacol.* 2002;53(6):641-643.

Erb JE, Erb TM. *The Slow Poisoning of America.* Virginia Beach, VA: Palladian Press; 2003.

He K, Du S, Xun P et al. Consumption of monosodium glutamate in relation to incidence of overweight in Chinese adults: China health and nutrition survey. *Am J Clin Nutr.* 2001;93(6):1328-1336.

Klotter J. MSG & obesity. *Townsend Letter for Doctors & Patients.* 2004 November; 256:17.

Meletis C. Cofactors and neurochemistry: the missing link for a healthy mind and body. *CPMedical.net.* http://www.cpmedical.net/articles/cofactors-and-neurochemistry-the-missing-link-for-a-healthy-mind-and-body. nd.

Mercola J. The shocking dangers of MSG you don't know. *Mercola.com.* http://articles.mercola.com/sites/articles/archive/2007/08/28/dangers-of-msg.aspx. Published August 28 2007.

Okiyama A, Beauchamp GK. Taste dimensions of MSG in a food system: role of glutamate in young American subjects. *Physiol Behav.* 1998;65(1):177-181.

Prescott J. Effects of added glutamate on liking for novel food flavors. *Appetite.* 2004;42(2):143-150.

Rogers PJ, Blundell JE. Umami and appetite: effects of monosodium glutamate on hunger and food intake in human subjects. *Physiol Behav.* 1990;48(6):801-804.

Sánchez-Villegas A, Toledo E, de Irala J, Ruiz-Canela M, Pla-Vidal J, Martínez-González MA. Fast-food and commercially baked goods consumption and the risk of depression. *Public Health Nutr.* 2012;15(3):424-432.

Williams AN, Woessner KM. Monosodium glutamate 'allergy': menace or myth? *Clin Exp Allergy.* 2009;39(5):640-646.

Yeomans MR, Gould NJ, Mobini S, Prescott J. Acquired flavor acceptance and intake facilitated by monosodium glutamate in humans. *Physiol Behav.* 2008;93(4-5):958-966.

Zarate CA Jr., Singh JB, Carlson PJ et al. A randomized trial of an N-methyl-D-aspartate antagonist in treatment-resistant major depression. *Arch Gen Psychiatry.* 2006;63(8):856-864.

Chapter 14 | Controlling Appetite with an UN-Diet

Beaumont, W. Nutrition Classics. Experiments and observations on the gastric juice and the physiology of digestion. By William Beaumont. Plattsburgh. Printed by F.P. Allen. 1833. *Nutr Rev.* 1977;35(6):144-145.

David M. *Nourishing Wisdom: A Mind-Body Approach to Nutrition and Well-Being.* New York, NY: Random House; 1991.

David M. *The Slow Down Diet: Eating for Pleasure, Energy and Weight Loss.* Rochester, VT: Healing Arts Press; 2005.

DeFina LF, Marcoux LG, Devers SM, Cleaver JP, Willis BL. Effects of omega-3 supplementation in combination with diet and exercise on weight loss and body composition. *Am J Clin Nutr.* 2011;93(2):455-462.

Greenblatt JM. *Answers to Anorexia: A Breakthrough Nutritional Treatment That Is Saving Lives.* North Branch, MN: Sunrise River Press; 2010.

Greenblatt JM. *The Breakthrough Depression Solution.* North Branch, MN: Sunrise River Press; 2011.

Guiliano M. *French Women Don't Get Fat.* New York, NY: Vintage Books; 2005.

Ross, J. *The Diet Cure.* New York, NY: Penguin Books; 1999.

Chapter 15 | Rediscovering Hope Through Therapy

Agras WS, Telch CF, Arnow B, Eldredge K, Marnell M. One-year follow-up of cognitive-behavioral therapy for obese individuals with binge eating disorder. *J Consult Clin Psychol.* 1997;65(2):343-347.

Amen D. ANT therapy: How to develop your own internal anteater to eradicate automatic negative thoughts. *AHHA.org.* http://www.ahha.org/articles.asp?Id=100. nd.

Ananth S. Developing healing beliefs. *Explore (NY).* 2009;5(6):354-355.

Bays, J. *Mindful eating: A guide to rediscovering a healthy and joyful relationship with food.* Boston, MA: Shambhala Publications; 2009.

Bougea AM, Spandideas N, Alexopoulos EC, Chrousos GP, Darviri C. Effect of the emotional freedom technique on perceived stress, quality of life and cortisol salivary levels in tension-type headache sufferers: a randomized controlled trial. *Explore (NY).* 2013;9(2):91-99.

Broderick PC. Mindfulness and coping with dysphoric mood: contrasts with rumination and distraction. *Cognit Ther Res.* 2005;29(5):501-510.

Butler LD, Symons BK, Henderson SL, Shortliffe LD, Spiegel D. Hypnosis reduces distress and duration of an invasive medical procedure for children. *Pediatrics.* 2005;115(1): e77-e85.

Center for Substance Abuse Treatment. *Substance abuse treatment: Group therapy. Treatment Improvement Protocol (TIP), 41.* Rockville, MD: Substance Abuse and Mental Health Services Administration (SAMHSA); 2005.

Church D, Yount G, Brooks AJ. The effect of emotional freedom techniques on stress biochemistry: a randomized controlled trial. *J Nerv Ment Dis.* 2012;200(10):891-896.

Devlin MJ, Goldfein JA, Petkova E, Liu L, Walsh BT. Cognitive behavioral therapy and fluoxetine for binge eating disorder: two-year follow-up. *Obes Res.* 2005;15(7):1077-1088.

Dodge E, Hodes M, Eisler T, Dare C. Family therapy for bulimia nervosa in adolescents: an exploratory study. *J Fam Ther.* 1995; 17:59-77.

Enea V, Dafinoiu I. Cognitive hypnotherapy in addressing the posttraumatic stress disorder. *Procedia Soc Behav Sci.* 2013;78(13):36-40.

Feinstein D. Energy psychology: a review of the preliminary evidence. *Psychotherapy (Chic).* 2008;45(2):199-213.

Feldman G. Cognitive and behavioral therapies for depression: overview, new directions and practical recommendations for dissemination. *Psychiatr Clin North Am.* 2007;30(1):39-50.

Grilo CM, Crosby RD, Wilson GT, Masheb RM. 2-month follow-up of fluoxetine and cognitive behavioral therapy for binge eating disorder. *J Consult Clin Psychol.* 2012;80(6):1108-13.

Gruzelier J. Theta synchronization of hippocampal and long distance circuitry in the brain: implications for EEG-Neurofeedback and hypnosis in the treatment of PTSD. In: Roy MJ, ed. *Novel Approaches to the Diagnosis and Treatment of Posttraumatic Stress Disorder.* Amsterdam, NLD: IOS Press; 2006: pp. 13-22.

Hutchinson-Phillips S, Jamieson GA, Gow K. Differing roles of imagination and hypnosis in self-regulation of eating behaviour. *Contemp Hypn.* 2005;22(4):171-183.

Johnson DL, Karkut RT. Participation in multicomponent hypnosis treatment programs for women's weight loss with and without overt aversion. *Psychol Rep.* 1996;79(2):659-668.

Kjaer TW, Bertelsen C, Piccini P, Brooks D, Alving J, Lou HC. Increased dopamine tone during meditation-induced change of consciousness. *Brain Res. Cogn Brain Res.* 2002;13(2):255-259.

Kristeller JL, Wolever RQ. Mindfulness-based eating awareness training for treating binge eating disorder: the conceptual foundation. *Eating Disord.* 2010;19(1):49-61.

Langer E. *Counterclockwise: Mindful health and the power of possibility.* New York, NY: Ballantine Books; 2009.

LeGrange D, Crosby RD, Rathrouz PJ, Leventhal BL. A randomized controlled comparison of family-based treatment and supportive psychotherapy for adolescents with bulimia nervosa. *Arch Gen Psychiatry.* 2007;64(9):1049-1056.

Lock J, LeGrange D. Family-based treatment of eating disorders. *Int J Eat Disord.* 2005;37(S1): S64-S67.

Lynch E. Emotional acupuncture. *Nurs Stand.* 2007;21(50):24-25.

McCaslin DL. A review of efficacy claims in energy psychology. *Psychotherapy (Chic)*. 2009;46(2):249-256.

Murphy R, Straebler S, Cooper Z, Fairburn CG. Cognitive behavioral therapy for eating disorders. *Psychiatr Clin North Am*. 2010;33(3):611-624.

Patterson DR, Jensen MP. Hypnosis and clinical pain. *Psychol Bull*. 2003;129(4):495-521.

Pendleton VR, Goodrick GK, Poston WS, Reeves RS, Foreyt JP. Exercise augments the effects of cognitive-behavioral therapy in the treatment of binge eating. *Int J Eat Disord*. 2002;31(2):172-184.

Pignotti M, Thyer B. Some comments on "Energy psychology: A review of the evidence": premature conclusions based on incomplete evidence? *Psychotherapy (Chic)*. 2009;46(2):257-261.

Poulsen S, Lunn S, Daniel SI et al. A randomized controlled trial of psychoanalytic psychotherapy or cognitive-behavioral therapy for bulimia nervosa. *Am J Psychiatry*. 2014;171(1):109-116.

Ray O. How the mind hurts and heals the body. *Am Psychol*. 2004;59(1):29-40.

Ricca V, Castellini G, Lo Sauro C, Rotella CM, Faravelli C. Zonisamide combined with cognitive behavioral Therapy in binge eating disorder: a one-year follow-up study. *Psychiatry*. 2009;6(11), 23-28.

Shedler J. The efficacy of psychodynamic psychotherapy. *Am Psychol*. 2010;65(2):98-109.

Sojcher R, Gould Fogerite S, Perlman A. Evidence and potential mechanisms for mindfulness practices and energy psychology for obesity and binge-eating disorder. *Explore (NY)*. 2012;8(5):271-276.

Spiegel D. Tranceformations: hypnosis in brain and body. *Depress Anxiety*. 2013;30(4):342-352.

Stein J. Charlie Sheen claims AA has a 5% success rate—is he right? *Los Angeles Times*. http://articles.latimes.com/2011/mar/03/news/la-heb-sheen-aa-20110302. Published March 3 2011.

Sundgot-Borgen J, Rosenvinge JH, Bahr R, Schneider LS. The effect of exercise, cognitive therapy and nutritional counseling in treating bulimia nervosa. *Med Sci Sports Exerc*. 2002;34(2):190-195.

Tahiri M, Mottillo S, Joseph L, Pilote L, Eisenberg MJ. Alternative smoking cessation aids: a meta-analysis of randomized controlled trials. *Am J Med.* 2012;125(6):576-584.

Trotzky AS. The treatment of eating disorders as addiction among adolescent females. *Int J Adolesc Med Health.* 2002;14(4):269-274.

Vella-Zarb RA, Mills JS, Westra HA, Carter JC, Keating L. A randomized controlled trial of motivational interviewing+self-help versus psychoeducation+self-help for binge eating. *Int J Eat Disord.* 2014;48(3):328-332.

Chapter 16 | Mastering the Balance of Movement and Sleep

Brondel L, Romer MA, Nougues PM, Touyarou P, Davenne D. Acute partial sleep deprivation increases food intake in healthy men. *Am J Clin Nutr.* 2010;91(6):1550–1559.

Broom DR, Batterham RL, King JA, Stensel DJ. Influence of resistance and aerobic exercise on hunger, circulating levels of acylated ghrelin and peptide YY in healthy males. *Am J Physiol.* 2009;296(1): R29-35.

Buchowski MS, Meade NN, Charboneau E et al. Aerobic Exercise training reduces cannabis craving and use in non-treatment seeking cannabis-dependent adults. *PLoS ONE.* 2011;6(3): e17465.

Calogero RM, Pedrotty KN. The practice and process of healthy exercise: An investigation of the treatment of exercise abuse in women with eating disorders. *Eat Disord.* 2004;12(4):273-291.

Cameron J, Doucet E. Getting to the bottom of feeding behavior: who's on top? *Appl Physiol Nutr Metab.* 2007;32(2):177-189.

Cappuccio FP, Taggart FM, Kandala NB et al. Meta-analysis of short sleep duration and obesity in children and adults. *Sleep.* 2010;31(5):619-626.

Catenacci VA, Ogden LG, Stuht J et al. Physical activity patterns in the national weight control registry. *Obesity.* 2008;16(1):153-161.

Chaouloff F. Physical exercise and brain monoamines: a review. *Acta Physiol Scand.* 1989;137(1):1-13.

Costin C. *The Eating Disorder Sourcebook*. Los Angeles, CA: Lowell House; 1996.

Crujeiras AB, Goyenechea E, Abete I et al. Weight regain after diet-induced loss is predicted by higher baseline leptin and lower ghrelin plasma levels. *J Clin Endocrinol Metab*. 2010;95(11):5037-44.

Dalle Grave R, Calugi S, Marchesini G. Compulsive exercise to control shape or weight in eating disorders: prevention, associated features and treatment outcomes. *Compr Psychiatry*. 2008;49(4):346-352.

Dallman MF. Stress-induced obesity and the emotional nervous system. *Trends Endocrinol Metab*. 2010;21(3):159-165.

DeBoar LB, Tart CD, Presnell KE, Powers MB, Baldwin AS, Smits JA. Physical activity as a moderator of the association between anxiety sensitivity and binge eating. *Eat Behav*. 2012;13(3):194-201.

Gardner A, Boles RG. Mitochondrial energy depletion in depression with somatization. *Psychother Psychom*. 2008;77(2):127-129.

Goodwin RD. Association between physical activity and mental disorders among adults in the United States. *Prev Med*. 2003;36(6):698–703.

Gout B, Bourges C, Paineau-Dubreuil S. Satiereal, a Crocus sativus L extract, reduces snacking and increases satiety in a randomized placebo-controlled study of mildly overweight, healthy women. *Nutr Res*. 2010;30(5):305-313.

Greer SM, Goldstein AN, Walker MP. The impact of sleep deprivation on food desire in the human brain. *Nat Commun*. 2013; 4:2259.

Harris AH, Cronkite R, Moos R. Physical activity, exercise coping and depression in a 10-year cohort study of depressed patients. *J Affect Disord*. 2006;93(1-3):79–85.

Harvey SB, Hotopf M, Overland S, Mykletun A. Physical activity and common mental disorders. *Br J Psychiatry*. 2010;197(5):357–364.

Imbeault P, Saint-Pierre S, Alméras N, Tremblay A. Acute effects of exercise on energy intake and feeding behaviour. *Br J Nutr*. 1997;77(4):511-21.

Khalsa SB, Shorter SM, Cope S, Wyshak G, Sklar E. Yoga ameliorates performance anxiety and mood disturbance in young professional musicians. *Appl Psychophysiol Biofeedback*. 2009;34(4):279–289.

King NA, Burley VJ, Blundell JE. Exercise-induced suppression of appetite: effects on food intake and implications for energy balance. *Eur J Clin Nutr.* 1994;48(10):715-274.

King NA, Caudwell PP, Hopkins M, Stubbs JR, Naslund E, Blundell JE. Dual-process action of exercise on appetite control: increase in orexigenic drive but improvement in meal-induced satiety. *Am J Clin Nutr.* 2009;90(4):921-927.

King NA, Tremblay A, Blundell JE. Effects of exercise on appetite control: implications for energy balance. *Med Sci Sports Exerc.* 1997;29(8):1076-1089.

Lawlor DA, Hopker SW. The effectiveness of exercise as an intervention in the management of depression: systematic review and meta-regression analysis of randomized controlled trials. *BMJ.* 2001;322(7289):763-767.

Levine MD, Marcus MD, Moulton P. Exercise in the treatment of binge eating disorder. *Int J Eat Disord.* 1996;19(2):171-177.

Markwald RR, Melanson EL, Smith MR et al. Impact of insufficient sleep on total daily energy expenditure, food intake and weight gain. *Proc Natl Acad Sci U S A.* 2013;110(14):5695–5700.

Martins C, Morgan LM, Bloom SR, Robertson M. Effects of exercise on gut peptides, energy intake and appetite. *J Endocrinol.* 2007;193(2):251-258.

Martins C, Robertson MD, Morgan LM. Effects of exercise and restrained eating behaviour on appetite control. *Proc Nutr Soc.* 2008;67(1):28-41.

Martins C, Truby H, Morgan LM. Short-term appetite control in response to a 6-week exercise programme in sedentary volunteers. *Br J Nutr.* 2007;98(4):834-842.

Mayer J, Roy P, Mitra KP. Relation between caloric intake, body weight and physical work: studies in an industrial male population in West Bengal. *Am J Clin Nutr.* 1956;4(2):169-175.

Nedeltcheva AV, Kilkus JM, Imperial J, Kasza K, Schoeller DA, Penev PD. Sleep curtailment is accompanied by increased intake of calories from snacks. *Am J Clin Nutr.* 2009;89(1):126-133.

Oh H, Taylor AH. Brisk walking reduces ad libitum snacking in regular chocolate eaters during a workplace simulation. *Appetite.* 2011;58(1):387-392.

Rezin GT, Amboni G, Zugno AI, Quevedo J, Streck EL. Mitochondrial dysfunction and psychiatric disorders. *Neurochem Res.* 2009;34(6):1021-1029.

Rice B, Janssen I, Hudson R, Ross R. Effects of aerobic or resistance exercise and/or diet on glucose tolerance and plasma insulin levels in obese men. *Diabetes Care.* 1999;22(5):684-691.

Spiegel K, Tasali E, Penev P, Van Cauter E. Brief communication: Sleep curtailment in healthy young men is associated with decreased leptin levels, elevated ghrelin levels and increased hunger and appetite. *Ann Intern Med.* 2004;141(11):846–850.

Srikanthan P, Karlamangla AA. Relative muscle mass is inversely associated with insulin resistance and prediabetes. Findings from the third national health and nutrition examination survey. *J Clin Endocrinol Metab.* 2011;96(9):2898-2903.

Tsatsoulis A, Fountoulakis S. The protective role of exercise on stress system dysregulation and comorbidities. *Ann N Y Acad Sci.* 2006; 1083:196-213.

Unick JL, Otto AD, Goodpaster BH, Helsel DL, Pellegrini CA, Jakcic JM. Acute effect of walking on energy intake in overweight/obese women. *Appetite.* 2010;55(3):413-419.

Van Cauter, E, Holmback U, Knutson K et al. Impact of sleep and sleep loss on neuroendocrine and metabolic function. *Horm Res.* 2007;67(Suppl 1):2-9.

PART V: YOUR NEW HOPE

Chapter 17 | Survival of the Fattest

Van der Laan LN, de Ridder DT, Viergever MA, Smeets PA. The first taste is always with the eyes: a meta-analysis on the neural correlates of processing visual food cues. *Neuroimage.* 2011;55(1):296-303.

Wang GJ, Volkow ND, Thanos PK, Fowler JS. Imaging of brain dopamine pathways: implications for understanding obesity. *J Addict Med.* 2009;3(1):8-18.

Psychiatry Redefined

Book Series

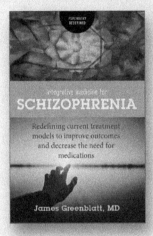
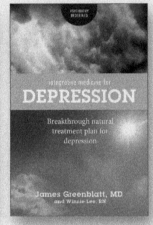
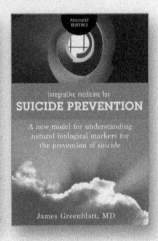
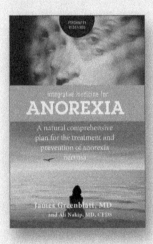
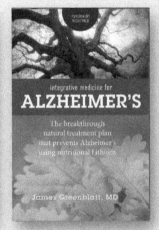
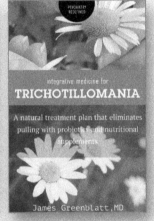

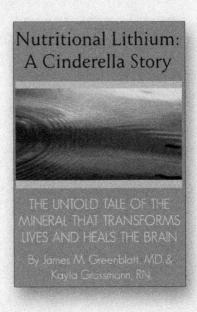
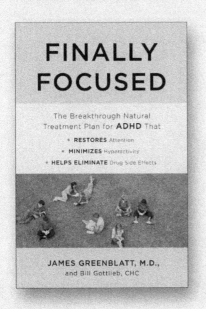
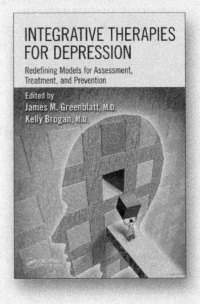

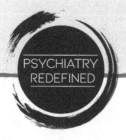

We Can Do Better

It is no secret that the current symptomatic treatment model of mental illness is not supporting our patients in recovery or wellness.

The field of psychiatry has lagged far behind in understanding the value of integrative medicine in the treatment of mental illness. This lag has created a wedge between patients and their healthcare providers.

Psychiatry Redefined acts as a bridge between patients and their healthcare providers, family members, and caregivers, that widens the possibilities of treating and sustaining mental health.

Psychiatry Redefined is a vision for mental health professionals, patients, family, and caregivers.

Psychiatry Redefined is dedicated to patients suffering from ineffective treatments, exhausted by their experience, and seeking more individualized care.

We Have To Do Better

James Greenblatt, MD

Please visit our website for more information

WWW.PSYCHIATRYREDEFINED.ORG

CPSIA information can be obtained
at www.ICGtesting.com
Printed in the USA
BVHW031024240720
584409BV00005B/373